Beth Shaw's YogaFit®

Beth Shaw

Human Kinetics

Library of Congress Cataloging-in-Publication Data

Shaw, Beth, 1966-
  [YogaFit]
  Beth Shaw's YogaFit / Beth Shaw.
    p. cm.
  ISBN 0-7360-3337-8
    1. Physical fitness.   2. Yoga, Hatha.   I. Title.
  RA781.7 .S446   2000
  613.7'046--dc21   00-056731

ISBN: 0-7360-3337-8

Acquisitions Editor: Martin Barnard; **Managing Editor**: Leigh LaHood; **Assistant Editor**: Kim Thoren; **Copyeditor**: Lisa Morgan; **Proofreader**: Joanna Hatzopoulos; **Graphic Designer**: Robert Reuther; **Graphic Artist**: Sandra Meier; **Cover Designer**: Jack W. Davis; **Photographer (cover and interior)**: Tom Roberts; **Printer**: Versa Press

Human Kinetics books are available at special discounts for bulk purchase. Special editions or book excerpts can also be created to specification. For details, contact the Special Sales Manager at Human Kinetics.

Printed in the United States of America   10   9   8   7   6   5   4   3   2   1

Human Kinetics
Web site: www.humankinetics.com

United States: Human Kinetics
P.O. Box 5076, Champaign, IL 61825-5076
800-747-4457
e-mail: humank@hkusa.com

Canada: Human Kinetics
475 Devonshire Road Unit 100, Windsor, ON N8Y 2L5
800-465-7301 (in Canada only)
e-mail: hkcan@mnsi.net

Europe: Human Kinetics
P.O. Box IW14, Leeds LS16 6TR, United Kingdom
+44 (0) 113 278 1708
e-mail: humank@hkeurope.com

Australia: Human Kinetics
57A Price Avenue, Lower Mitcham, South Australia 5062
08 8277 1555
e-mail: liahka@senet.com.au

New Zealand: Human Kinetics
P.O. Box 105-231, Auckland Central
09-309-1890
e-mail: hkp@ihug.co.nz

For all of my friends and family,
students, teachers, and coworkers:
thank you for supporting the vision
and helping make the dream a reality.
Namasté!

Contents

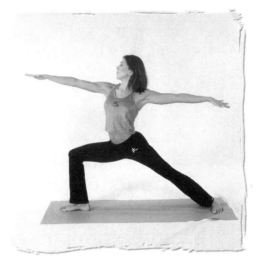

PART I   YogaFit Poses . . . 1

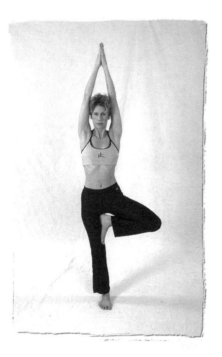

PART II YogaFit Workouts . . . 131

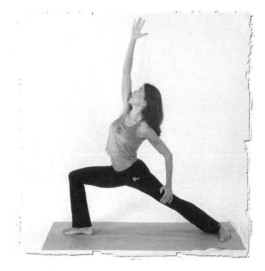

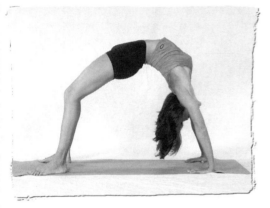

Pose Index

Preface

As we enter the new millennium, the hottest fitness trend is one of the oldest fitness practices—yoga. Why? Because modern athletes and fitness participants are increasingly aware that peak performance requires focus and coordination from both the body and the mind.

Unfortunately, many popular myths about yoga have inhibited people from enthusiastically embracing it. These myths include the following: yoga does not give you a real workout; yoga's ancient roots and spiritual associations conflict with modern lifestyles; and yoga involves a lot of mumbo-jumbo, including weird Sanskrit names for the exercises. Sound about right? Then you should try YogaFit!

YogaFit is an effective and exciting workout program for physically active people that balances body and mind, gets you into great shape, focuses your effort, and helps prevent sports injuries. YogaFit includes the elements of a tough cardiovascular workout as well as strength-building yoga poses that lengthen and strengthen your muscles without adding unnecessary bulk. Pretty much what contemporary sports-fitness physicians prescribe. YogaFit also helps you choose the right setting and the right music for your specific yoga experience so you can really lose yourself in the practice, release stress and tension, and totally focus on building mental strength and terrific body tone.

If you're still feeling a little hesitant, I understand. Most of us who have contemplated taking traditional yoga classes have been intimidated by images of yogis in pretzel poses (actually, you will find yourself able to perform some of these poses yourself sooner and more easily than you might think), or we've encountered yoga teachers who appeared unapproachable, sometimes even otherworldly. It's not surprising that, given these images and the myths I mentioned earlier, yoga often seems to be reserved for an elite group of people: ultra-flexible individuals, vegetarians, and those who have studied for decades with yogis from India who chant!

Of course, there's nothing wrong with being ultra-flexible or vegetarian, knowing how to chant, going to India, or being fluent in Sanskrit. Certain elements of yoga hold some fascination for some of us, but many of these traditions can, understandably, also make us uncomfortable. Personally, I feel a deep respect and admiration for the ancient tradition of yoga and all traditional yogis and practitioners. After all, they taught me about the necessity of coordinating body and mind. They got me started. They got me hooked. But once I started teaching, I quickly learned that the popular prejudices against traditional yoga stopped many people from trying it, and that most people, particularly athletes and serious fitness buffs, were not prepared to change their lives or lifestyles to obtain the benefits of yoga.

Well, the truth is, you don't have to change your life; and if you are already serious about fitness, either professionally or simply because being fit is an integral part of your daily routine, you won't have to change your lifestyle, either! (Obviously, if you are new to fitness and you have a lifestyle that is not currently supporting your health, you will have to change things a bit, just as you would for any fitness development program.) I created YogaFit to fulfill the needs of athletic and fit people like myself who want to enrich their workouts with exercises guaranteed to focus minds and trim and tone bodies. YogaFit is a program for everyone, and bringing this program to you is what makes YogaFit an exciting and rewarding journey for me!

There are a few basic principles that are the foundation of a YogaFit workout. First of all, it should be understood that the word *workout* is used in its literal sense. YogaFit makes you sweat—profusely at times—and work pretty hard. It combines aerobic and anaerobic movements, as well as elements of hatha yoga, with traditional exercise. After a YogaFit workout, you will feel you have done something good for your body.

YogaFit is about exploring your limits, physically and mentally; it is the ultimate mind-working-with-muscle challenge. You will learn how to stay relaxed in demanding physical situations, and you will be able to transfer this skill to other aspects of your life. Your muscles will store memories that can be triggered when you need to relax in all kinds of stressful situations, physically and emotionally. Think of YogaFit as a form of preventive medicine—a complete body/mind workout for fitness-oriented people.

After regular YogaFit workouts, you will experience increased strength and stamina, natural weight loss, a higher energy level, more vitality, longer and leaner muscles, and better body tone. You will also have more body awareness, increased inner strength, better concentration, an improved self-image, more self-confidence and will power, and a certain inner peace and tranquility, all of which will result in noticeable stress reduction.

What separates YogaFit from other forms of yoga is that YogaFit speaks directly and without any pretentiousness to everyone, but especially to the needs of amateur and professional athletes. You know that to be successful, you need to avoid or prevent injury. You know that your mind can trick you out of exercising efficiently (or exercising at all) on a regular basis. You know that your favorite sport or discipline stresses only certain body parts and that you need to balance your body to be in really great shape. YogaFit holds the answers to all of these problems without boring you to death.

Another of my goals is to package the YogaFit workout in a format that is sensual—a format that appeals to the senses of sight, touch, smell, and hearing. The YogaFit workout is designed to excite you and capture your imagination. YogaFit means sweat, movement, great music, dimmed lights, and stimulating smells. You will always want to come back for more.

So let's make a pact. You bring the commitment to practice regularly (no cheating), and I will give you all the necessary tools to assemble your very own customized YogaFit workouts. My promise is that the results will be visible within a few weeks—and the benefits will be lifelong if you continue to practice these exercises.

In this book I will teach you 53 basic YogaFit poses, and I will show you how to assemble them into well-rounded YogaFit workouts that can be modified to serve your personal needs and purposes at different times. I will also explain how to use YogaFit as a cross-training practice with other sports. Whether you are a professional athlete seeking to balance your workout routine, an avid visitor to the gym looking for a new challenge, or an infrequent exerciser striving to reach a higher level of fitness, this book will help you achieve your goals. YogaFit can be a challenging workout in your life, whether you have prior yoga experience or not.

I developed YogaFit over the past decade after completing several yoga certifications. Because of my background in the fitness industry, I saw the need to bring yoga to the masses via the health club environment. Since the creation of YogaFit, my staff and I have trained thousands of YogaFit teachers in fitness facilities worldwide. My personal mission with YogaFit is to contribute to society by sharing the gift of yoga. Participants in our Teacher Training program must devote eight hours of community service teaching to a group of participants who normally would not have the opportunity to receive it. We also host charitable fundraisers in our signature YogaFit studio in Hermosa Beach.

YogaFit is the miracle in my life. Bringing my vision of a user-friendly and totally accessible form of yoga to a broad audience who can share its incredible benefits is an extraordinarily rewarding experience. You just found the workout of the new millennium. Have fun with this book, and make YogaFit the miracle in your life!

What Is YogaFit?

created YogaFit in 1994. YogaFit combines elements of hatha yoga with traditional fitness exercises and stretching routines.

YogaFit is a hybrid yoga specifically designed for athletes and the mainstream fitness industry. YogaFit integrates body and mind for total performance, and it is therefore an effective means of achieving body/mind health. YogaFit features both strength and conditioning components, and it uses contemporary music to enhance the experience.

YogaFit was created to provide individual athletes, sport teams, fitness enthusiasts, sport centers, and gyms with a ready-made yoga program that is appropriate for all ages and fitness levels. YogaFit is a demystified yoga program that is affordable, easy to learn, and conveniently accessible.

The YogaFit Concept

YogaFit appeals to athletes and fitness enthusiasts because it provides them with a balanced, total body/mind workout. *Workout* meaning we sweat and build strength without strain or bulk. *Balanced* meaning we work all muscle groups evenly in each session. *Body/mind* meaning we also work the mental muscle to increase willpower, determination, and ultimately endurance. As an athlete, you will notice that a regular YogaFit workout will give you incredible muscle tone, increased flexibility, and better overall health and fitness, which will lead to a lower risk of injuries and chronic pain.

By focusing inward and working with your breath, you will dramatically improve your body awareness. This will help you to make all of your athletic activities more meaningful and efficient. It will also help you understand your physical limitations and your mental boundaries. You will learn that your mind often is the only thing holding you back from peak performance, and you will understand how to better overcome your mental hang-ups by listening to and understanding your body.

Although based on an ancient Indian practice, YogaFit does not adhere to a particular philosophy, religion, or type of meditation. I understood that the "cult" aspect of traditional yoga was one of the main reasons why yoga did not appeal to bigger numbers of people in the past. YogaFit is cult-free, and your lifestyle remains your business.

YogaFit demystifies yoga. Based on the proven benefits of a yoga practice, the YogaFit workout is simple and systematic. In YogaFit we use English, not Sanskrit names for all poses. We do not chant, but we work so hard that we can feel the sweat drip off our bodies. We are not necessarily vegetarians, nor do we lead "spiritual" lifestyles, but we still enjoy working with our bodies and our minds at the same time. I do not believe that the ancient secrets of yoga and all its wonderful benefits are only accessible to those who have practiced for at least a decade; I take the ancient wisdom and put it into the 21st century, into Western culture, to fit people's needs today. I want as many people as possible to enjoy the wonderful benefits of a great yoga workout.

YogaFit is easy to learn and easy to teach. Anyone with a health- or fitness-related background and a good working knowledge of anatomy and biomechanics can learn the YogaFit system. We have taught thousands to teach fun and effective yoga classes with our training program. In fact, at YogaFit we spend more time teaching our teachers than any major fitness certification program, and although we are the only IHRSA (International Health, Racquet and Sportsclub Association), ACE (American Council on Exercise), and AFAA (Aerobics and Fitness Association of America) approved yoga teacher training program, our training fee is only a fraction of what it is for other yoga teacher training programs. Our goal is to train as many teachers as possible, because we see how wonderfully YogaFit affects the lives of those it touches.

YogaFit is perfect for group training, and it can be combined with any other sport for cross-training and performance-enhancing purposes. You can find more details on this aspect of YogaFit in chapter 11.

YogaFit Versus Traditional Yoga

Although there is no need for you to become an expert on the subject of yoga, you should be aware of the integral differences between yoga and YogaFit. The following comparison chart will help you better understand the purpose of a YogaFit workout and the philosophy behind this contemporary body/mind workout.

Traditional Yoga	YogaFit
Six-thousand-year-old science that originated in India	Demystified, contemporary yoga for mainstream fitness enthusiasts
Designed to ready the body for meditation	Designed for athletes and fitness enthusiasts
Styles	**Styles**
Hatha yoga—includes all physical yoga, such as the following types	YogaFit®
Ashtanga yoga—uses a sequence of specific and mostly advanced poses	Power YogaFit®
Kundalini yoga—focuses on bringing energy to the body and on deep rhythmic breathing	YogaFit® Lite
Iyengar yoga—stresses alignment and perfecting poses that are held for long periods; uses props	Pre/Postnatal YogaFit®
Restorative yoga—favors the use of props for supported poses; ideal for injured people and those desiring relaxation	
Involves	**Does NOT involve**
Chanting, Sanskrit words, religious disciplines	Chanting, Sanskrit words, religious disciplines
Purpose	**Purpose**
To bring together various aspects of the self	To provide the best body/mind workout ever

The Benefits of YogaFit

A regular YogaFit workout gives you all the benefits of a traditional yoga practice and more. Best results are achieved by practicing at least three times a week for 45 to 60 minutes each time. Here are the most common results, which can be visible very soon after you start your YogaFit practice. But remember, the longer and more consistently you practice, the more you will benefit from YogaFit.

- Increased flexibility
- Stronger muscles
- Better body tone
- Elongated muscles without bulk
- Relaxed and clear mind
- Reduced stress
- Increased body awareness
- Natural weight loss
- Improved posture
- Strengthened immune system

In addition to the benefits of a traditional yoga practice, a regular YogaFit workout will also help you specifically in your athletic endeavors in the following ways:

- Helps prevent injuries by keeping your muscles supple
- Supports a more effective metabolic exchange during all physical activities by teaching better breathing patterns
- Balances unevenness of other workouts by supplying a total body/mind workout that works all muscle groups
- Increases endurance, willpower, and discipline by working not only your body but also your mind

Please see chapter 11 for more information on how to use YogaFit to effectively cross-train with your favorite sports.

YogaFit Workout Essentials

The beauty of a YogaFit workout lies not only in its many benefits but also in the fact that it will probably be the easiest and least expensive workout you have ever started. No expensive equipment or gear is needed. Here are some recommendations for making your YogaFit workouts as pleasurable as possible.

Clothing

Wear comfortable workout clothes. I do not recommend baggy clothing, because it will be obstructive during your workout. Wearing layers of fitted clothing is a big advantage; you can start out wearing long sleeves and then pare down to just a tank top or bra top when your body has heated up. Both long pants and shorts are fine. Make your own personal choices. For the cool-down or deep relaxation, I recommend that you cover up again. And don't forget—no shoes, no socks. YogaFit is best practiced barefoot.

Mats

The one thing I urge you to purchase as soon as possible is a high-quality yoga mat. Decide for yourself if you prefer a thick or thin mat. All yoga mats are sticky so that you and your mat won't slide along the floor. There are some extra-long yoga mats on the market that give you more space.

Props

YogaFit is best practiced on a wooden floor with your mat. Should you have sensitive knees, you might consider getting a knee pad, which lies on top of your mat to protect your knees during kneeling poses. If you have tight shoulders, like many athletes, you should get a shoulder strap. This will help you get all the benefits out of shoulder-opening poses (most important, it will allow you to get into the poses in the first place). For tight hamstrings, get blocks, which allow you to hold the proper alignment in certain poses. (See part I for a description of the proper use of these props.)

Workout Video

YogaFit and Human Kinetics have published a brand-new YogaFit workout video, titled *Beth Shaw's YogaFit Workout*, that leads you through an actual YogaFit workout. This video can help you get started with a regular YogaFit practice. It shows you what you need for your workout, what the YogaFit pros wear, how they move from pose to pose, and what the poses should look like.

Music

I like to listen to some inspiring and motivating music during YogaFit workouts, so I have compiled YogaFit sampler CDs containing my favorite tunes. These CDs lead you through a total one-hour YogaFit workout. For more information, see **www.yogafit.com**. Of course, you can also use your personal favorites.

Where to Buy

YogaFit sells all the items just mentioned—hot and sexy as well as practical and comfortable clothing, mats, knee pads, shoulder straps, blocks, workout video, music CDs, and more (audiotapes, audio CDs). You can contact YogaFit at 888-786-3111 or 310-798-8773, or you can purchase online at **www.yogafit.com**. To order more copies of this book or a copy of *Beth Shaw's YogaFit Workout* video, you can contact either YogaFit or Human Kinetics (**www.humankinetics.com** or 800-747-4457), or check with your local or online bookstore.

From here you should move on to the next section of this book, which explains the philosophy of YogaFit and the essence of the YogaFit practice in more detail. It also gives you some important information on how seniors, children, pregnant women, and those with medical conditions should approach YogaFit.

PART I

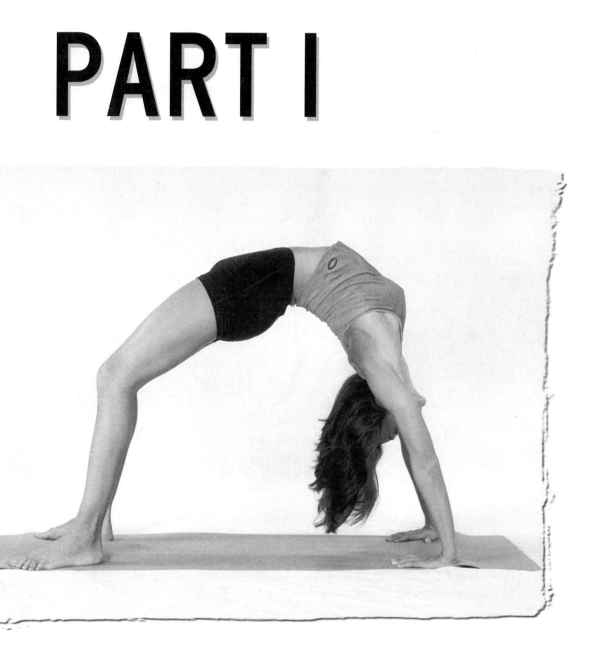

YogaFit Poses

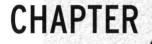

1

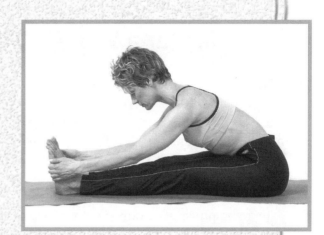

Starting With YogaFit

Before you start your yoga practice, make sure you are very familiar with this chapter. It covers the essence of YogaFit, how to prepare for class, the benefits of a regular YogaFit workout, and very important modifications for practitioners with special conditions and injuries.

Preparing for a YogaFit Workout

Follow these simple guidelines to maximize the beneficial effects and pleasure of your YogaFit practice.

Know your limits. Start your first YogaFit workout only after you read through this entire book, and possibly, after you have looked at the entire *Beth Shaw's YogaFit Workout* video. Be sure to check with your physician before starting this or any other new workout. This is especially important if you have any injuries or chronic illnesses or if you are pregnant, over 65, or in poor physical condition. In addition, read diligently through the "Special Conditions" section of this chapter on how to modify this workout for your special condition.

Take time to familiarize yourself with the YogaFit concept. Go slowly through your first workout. Go at your own pace. Stop and take breaks when you need them. Your body is different every day. Be aware of your body's needs and requirements before, during, and after any YogaFit practice. Know what's best for you in the moment and listen to your body at all times. There is no competition in yoga or YogaFit and there are no medals for the ones who do the most poses.

Allow at least an hour and a half between eating and your practice. Meals should be light and easy to digest. If you need a snack before class, it should be fruit, tea, or an energy drink.

Stop any other activity at least 15 minutes before each practice. Use that time to calm, collect, and center yourself. This is also a good time to prepare the room. Turn off (or tone down) harsh lighting. Light candles, preferably glass-enclosed and/or aromatherapy scented ones. Use inspiring music to create an atmosphere that helps you focus, and leave all the everyday thoughts behind you. Make sure you won't have to get up to change music during your workout.

Face away from mirrored walls. Roll out your mat in a space that will not restrict you in any of the poses (that is, don't be too close to walls, doors, or furniture).

Smile, and consciously try to release any holding patterns in your face, neck, and shoulders. Make any adjustments that seem right to you, and make this practice an enjoyable experience that you want to come back to often.

The Three Mountains of the YogaFit Workout

You will notice that each YogaFit workout has a special sequence to it. If you follow our class formats, you will come to understand the logic of it. Every YogaFit workout consists of three parts, or *mountains*:

- Mountain I: Warm-up (heat-building exercises)
- Mountain II: Work (more strenuous poses and flow series)
- Mountain III: Deep and relaxing stretches (hip openers, back bends, inversions, resting poses)

Mountain I starts with a few minutes of breathing exercises to help turn your concentration inward and to connect body and breath. It is essential to build enough heat during Mountains I and II to prepare for the deep stretches that follow. YogaFit workouts build heat with a series of rapidly flowing poses which provide an elevation in heart rate. Sweat is a desirable by-product of this class segment.

After adequate heat has built in Mountain I, we move to Mountain II, the work phase of the class. More complicated, complex, and challenging poses flow together through longer holds.

The deep stretching poses found in Mountain III help release the stress and tension that is frequently held in our muscles. Furthermore, the poses we do in this part of the class help lengthen and strengthen muscles for an amazing body tone and increased flexibility and vitality.

The last part of Mountain III consists of several minutes of deep relaxation. This segment of the class can be used for meditation and guided visualization and to help restore energy, decrease stress, and cool down the body.

The Essence of YogaFit

There is no wrong way of doing yoga or a YogaFit workout. It does not matter how deep you can go into each pose or whether you can attempt the pose as described in your first, second, or twenty-second workout. Each body is different on any given day, and it is up to each of us to respect our own limitations. We all have physical and mental weaknesses and strengths; in YogaFit it is important to observe our bodies in the workout without judging them. The following principles form the essence of YogaFit and should be applied during every YogaFit session to make your practice as meaningful as possible. These principles, and not competitiveness or vanity, should be the basis of your YogaFit workout.

Breathing

All YogaFit breathing is done through the nose only. As a general rule, we open up, or expand, the body on the inhale and fold, or contract, the body (except in the abdominal work) on the exhale. Deep, diaphragmatic breathing is the key to a successful practice. The breath is the most powerful tool we have to calm and relax our bodies and clear our minds. It also helps us to get into poses more deeply. The breath should flow naturally with the pose and be connected with the movement.

Feeling

Breathing and feeling are the pillars of a successful YogaFit practice. Listening to the body helps us understand limitations and prevent injuries. Becoming aware of how your body feels in each pose helps bring you to your personal limit.

Clear Mind

It is essential to turn your focus inward. Work with your eyes closed as much as possible. Avoid mirror gazing and comparing yourself with others. There is no competition in YogaFit, no judgment, and no expectations. YogaFit is a process designed to help each person become the best he or she can be. The focus lies in the breath and the movement with the breath to clear the mind of any incoming thoughts.

Things to Remember
- Be aware of your breathing.
- Tune in with your body.
- Be sensitive to your body.
- Give up expectations of what you "should" be able to do.
- Be noncompetitive.
- Don't judge yourself.

Guidance and Motivation

Now that you know the essence of YogaFit, you can use some or all of the following phrases to motivate yourself or others. Feel free to modify these motivational tidbits to your own needs, but make sure the essence remains.

Feel free to repeat these phrases out loud or form them in your mind as often as you like during your YogaFit workout. In the beginning it is a good idea to write down your favorite YogaFit phrases and keep the notes with you during your workout.

On Breathing

- Breathe only through the nose while moving.
- Bring the breath into the tight spots in the body.
- Focus on the breath to clear the mind.
- Sink deeper into the pose with each breath.
- Connect breath with movement.

On Feeling

- If you are feeling something, it's working.
- Find maximum sensation in each pose.
- Don't push yourself too hard. Know your limits.
- Check in with your body. Notice how you feel.

On Working Through the Poses

- Let go of competitiveness, judgment, and expectations.
- Use flowing, graceful movements.
- Don't let your mind limit your body.
- We are on a journey of the body and mind.
- Take a break if you need to—honor your body.
- Keep your mind clear and calm at all times.
- All movement originates from the center.
- Strong abdominals protect your back.

Physical and Mental Benefits of a YogaFit Workout

Physical exercise not only works our muscles but also triggers a variety of biochemical and physiological reactions. YogaFit, as a hybrid of yoga and exercise, confers a variety of physical and mental benefits and leads to improved health and vitality.

The most important benefits of a regular YogaFit practice (see the list that follows) can be observed after just one week if you practice 45 to 60 minutes, three to five times a week. This will give you a good jump start. Continue your regular practice for another week, and you will see these benefits further unfold. After this two-week intensive YogaFit training, you will feel familiar with the poses and the sequencing, and you'll see and feel how your body has started to change and your mind has become clearer. To keep the good work up, try to get in as many 45- to 60-minute workouts a week as you can, but never fall under three per week. You can split up the time, doing a 30-minute workout in the morning and 30-minute workout in the evening, but try to get in at least two full (45- to 60-minute) sessions per week.

Here are some of the most important benefits of regular (at least three times per week for 45 to 60 minutes) YogaFit workouts:

- Counteracts brain aging
- Minimizes physical effects of aging
- Dramatically improves muscle tone
- Visibly reduces stress
- Enhances willpower and determination
- Promotes natural weight loss
- Significantly improves posture
- Stimulates digestion naturally
- Improves overall health and vitality
- Strengthens the immune system

Note: We store many emotions and memories in our muscles that can be released during a YogaFit workout. For example, hip openers such as the Pigeon pose might trigger physical sensations or emotional reactions. Do not be alarmed if you cry or have an emotional release during a YogaFit workout. This is a natural part of yoga and the healing process. Do not react to anyone else's emotional release during class or try to "fix" the situation; you will only call more attention to it. All you can do is provide a safe, comfortable, nonjudgmental environment for yourself and others.

Just as you might experience an emotional release during a YogaFit class, you might also experience a physical release. A physical release might manifest in any of the following ways:

- Tingling sensations
- Mild nausea

- Dizziness
- Light-headedness

In time, these sensations should pass. If they occur, take it easy or just rest. If you choose to continue with the practice, go slowly until the sensation passes.

Be assured that these physical reactions are not uncommon and are a natural way for the body to release stress and tension. Not everyone experiences physical or emotional release in these forms. Observe how your body reacts to the YogaFit practice without making any judgments.

Special Conditions

YogaFit students must take special care and modify their practices for any pertinent special conditions such as pregnancy, injury, or any medical condition. Inverted poses and back bends are for advanced students after intense warm-up only. Women who are menstruating should avoid inverted poses. Inversions reverse the natural flow of the menstruation and possibly promote endomitriosis.

Injuries or Medical Conditions

Here is a list of some common injuries and medical conditions and the appropriate modifications that need to be made to the YogaFit workout as a result.

Sciatica: Avoid forward bends without slight bend in the knees, or intense hamstring stretching.

Hypertension or high blood pressure: Avoid breath retention and inverted postures.

Glaucoma or other eye problems; ear congestion: Avoid breath retention and inverted postures.

Lower-back injuries: Bend the knees slightly during all types of forward folds to reduce the strain on the back.

Back or neck injuries: Avoid inverted postures.

Knee problems: Avoid quadriceps stretches such as the Camel pose and the Quad Stretch. Limit the use of the Pigeon pose. Place extra padding under the knees during floor work.

As a rule, people with special conditions should avoid the more intense or strenuous types of postures. Most postures can be modified (that is, made easier) and still provide beneficial effects.

Pregnancy

Although YogaFit is wonderful for prenatal conditioning, pregnant women should consult with their doctors before beginning, as they would for any exercise program.

Women who are used to performing regular exercise will experience a decline in performance during pregnancy. This is unavoidable, and pregnant women should not try to overcompensate for it. In fact, because there's less oxygen available for aerobic exercise, pregnant women *need* to limit the intensity of their workouts and to lower their target heart rates.

Pregnant women should avoid overstretching. Hormonal changes cause ligaments to loosen, and going too deep into a posture may result in injury. Pregnant women should also avoid lower spinal twists, lunges, forward bends, and spine-lying poses (for example, Spinal Twist—seated or lying down, Warrior poses, Forward Fold—seated or standing, or Child's Pose unless knees are apart). Prolonged inverted postures and breath retention should not be practiced, because these may limit the flow of blood to the fetus. In addition, pregnancy may affect circulation, so it's important to keep warm. After the first trimester, pregnant women should avoid prolonged periods of standing or lying flat on their backs. YogaFit poses can be modified to accommodate the physical changes in pregnant women's bodies. For example, in the third trimester, a wall or chair can be used to aid balance.

Body changes remain for four to six weeks after pregnancy. New mothers should be careful not to overextend themselves, and they should take their time to gradually work back into their regular YogaFit routines.

Age

YogaFit for seniors is based on simple, repetitive movements. Older yoga students can derive enormous benefits from such movements when they are combined with breathing techniques. In fact, the single most important point of focus in a YogaFit class for seniors is deep breathing.

If you are over 65, you should begin each workout with an extended warm-up period, as we do in our YogaFit classes for seniors, and you should take more time to focus on your breath and on balance. Some of the poses can be done sitting in a chair, and you can use a chair (or wall) for balance and support in the standing postures. At the end of your workout, allow at least 10 minutes for relaxation.

A YogaFit workout for seniors incorporates lots of shoulder openers to help improve posture. Shoulder-opening poses include those listed here:

- Standing Lateral Flexion
- Chest Expansion
- Knot pose
- Back Bends (after thorough warm-up)

The older yoga student should initially avoid some poses, including the following.

- Extended periods of inversion (especially for seniors with glaucoma or cataracts)
- Extended periods of floor postures and forward flexion
- Complex postures or those requiring a great deal of strength

Beginning Your Practice

Now that you know all about YogaFit and the YogaFit workout, it is time to get started with your first practice. Always come back to this chapter to review what YogaFit is all about and to deepen your knowledge. The more you know about YogaFit, and the more consistently you practice, the greater the benefits you will be able to receive.

CHAPTER

2

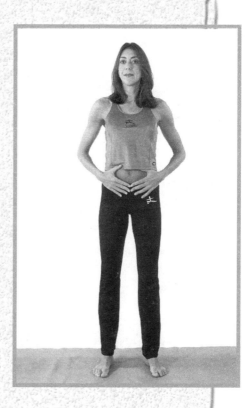

YogaFit
Breathing

n YogaFit we use various types of breathing. Understand the differences between them and apply the techniques accordingly.

Sinking Breath

Inhale, and feel your body lift slightly. Exhale, and let your body sink deeper into the pose.

Use the sinking breath with poses that move toward the center of the earth (e.g., the Forward Fold, the Downward Facing Dog, and the Chest Expansion).

Expanding Breath

Inhale, and feel your body expand and open up. Keep that open feeling while you exhale.

Use the expanding breath with poses that open to the sky (e.g., the Back Bend, the Triangle, and the Camel).

Three-Part Breath

Inhale, bring the breath deep into the abdomen, then fill the chest and ultimately the throat. Exhale, and let everything go.

Use the three-part breath when on your back at the beginning or end of class. It promotes deeper awareness of the breath. (See pages 16-17.)

Relaxation Breath

Inhale slowly (to the count of eight). Exhale slowly (to the count of eight). Repeat for one to two minutes. Remember to relax and feel the breath.

If necessary, you can gradually extend the length of your breath. (Inhale and exhale to the count of four for four or five breaths, progress to a count of six, then build to a count of eight or ten.)

Use the relaxation breath at the start or the end of class (i.e., during the warm-up or during final relaxation).

Breath of Fire

Sitting cross-legged, place your hands on your stomach. Inhale and exhale in short, rapid pulses. Feel the abdomen come in on each exhale. Maintain this rapid breath (10 to 20 times), then hold the breath. Bring your chin down, and feel the heat rise in your body. Repeat this sequence three times.

Use the breath of fire to create heat in the body (on colder days and when your energy level is low).

THREE-PART BREATH

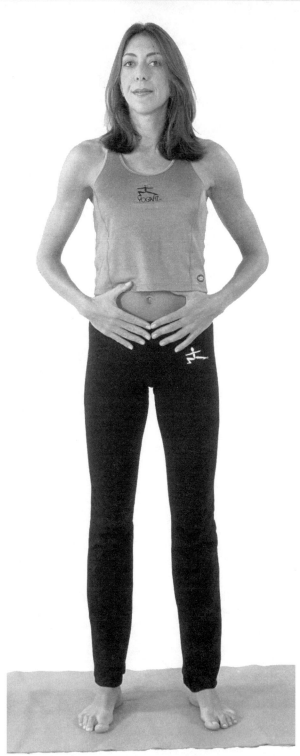

THREE-PART BREATH

Strengthens: Lungs • Abdominals

Use the Three-Part Breath at the start of every class (for five minutes). Benefits of this breath include stress reduction and greater body and breath awareness.

Getting into the pose

The Three-Part Breath can be done lying down or standing. Place your hands flat on your midsection.

Holding the pose

Breathe deeply through the nose. Feel the abdomen fill on the inhalation and contract on the exhalation. Focus on your posture and on proper alignment. Relax your shoulders and contract your abs.

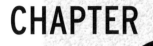

CHAPTER

3

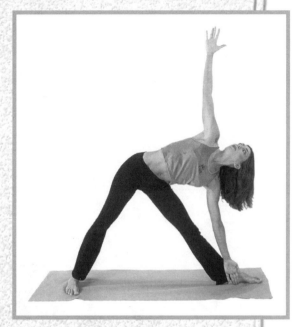

Standing and Balancing Poses

MOUNTAIN POSE

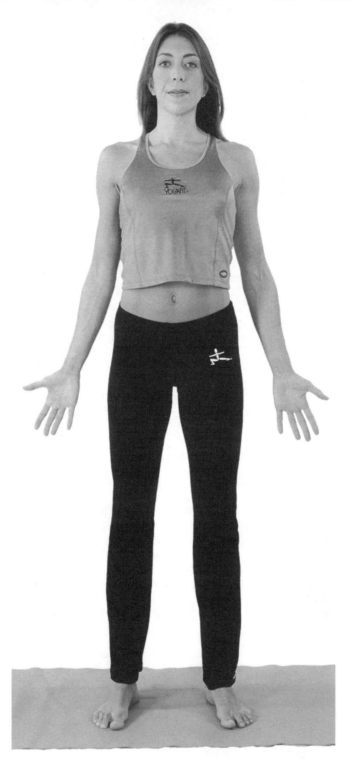

MOUNTAIN POSE

Use this pose at the beginning, middle, or end of practice, to check in with the body. It increases awareness of the body and the breath.

Getting into the pose

Stand straight, with your arms at your sides and your feet hip-width apart. Bend your knees slightly, keep your spine straight, and bring your shoulders back and away from the ears. Lift your chest slightly, tighten your abs, tuck your tail bone, and tighten the glutes.

Holding the pose

Breathe deeply into the chest. Relax your shoulders, close your eyes, and "go inside."

STANDING LATERAL FLEXION

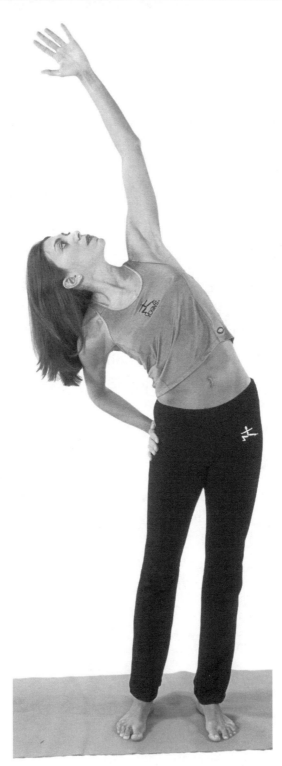

STANDING LATERAL FLEXION

 Strengthens: Waist
Stretches: Latissimus dorsi • Obliques • Major back
muscles

This pose is good to assume between standing poses,
during Mountain I or Mountain II. It is a side-opening pose.

Getting into the pose

Lift your arms over your head. Extend up from the navel
center. Lower one arm down to the side of your leg, and
slide your upper body down to that side.

Holding the pose

Breathe into your sides, rib cage, waist, and chest. Keep
proper alignment. Don't let your upper body fall forward.
Come up and switch sides.

CHAIR AND BALANCE CHAIR

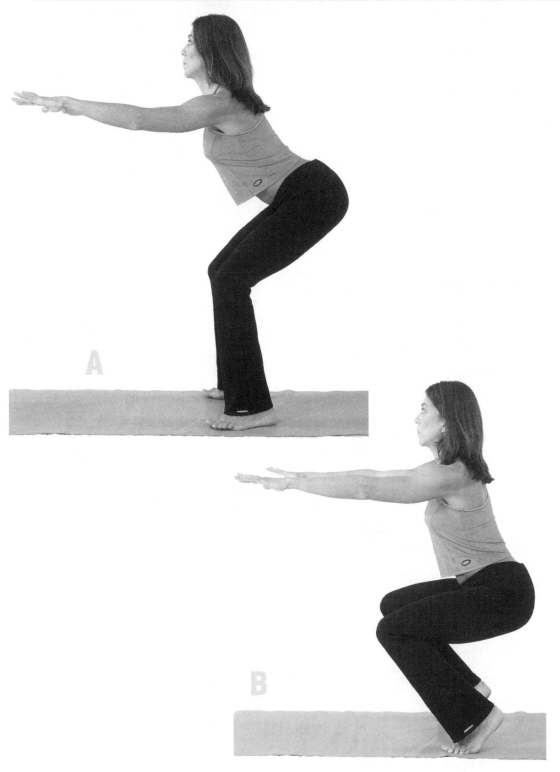

A

B

CHAIR AND BALANCE CHAIR

 Strengthens: Quads • Glutes • Feet and ankles

Use the Chair and Balance Chair poses to build heat and strength and to warm up the lower body, during Mountain I or Mountain II.

Getting into the pose

As if you are sitting in a chair, bend your knees and drop your buttocks (A).

Holding the pose

Push your tailbone back. Lift your chest to the sky. Lift your arms parallel to the floor, elbows slightly bent. Breathe into your navel center. Drop and relax your shoulders. Keep your knees behind your toes.

Balance Chair

Advanced pose: Come up on your toes and sit a bit lower (B). Find a focal point and breathe.

Modification

People with foot problems should be careful on their toes.

WARRIOR I

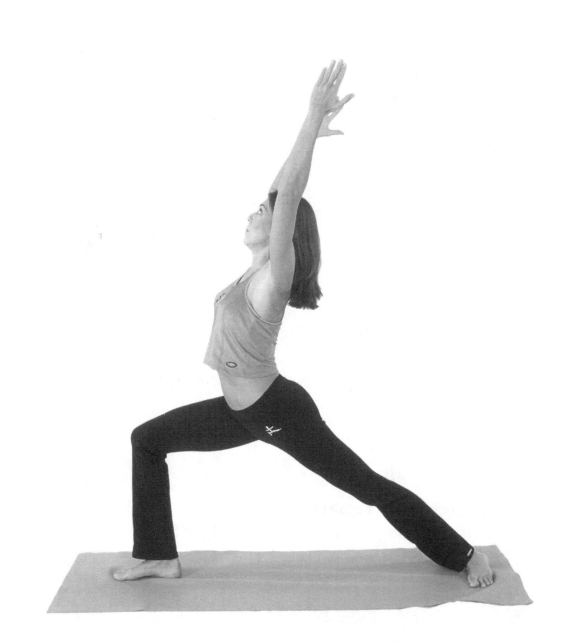

WARRIOR I

 Strengthens: Quads • Glutes • Upper body
Stretches: Lats • Hip flexors

This pose is part of the Warrior series. Benefits include increased physical and mental strength and enhanced willpower and determination. Use it during Mountain II.

Getting into the pose

Step your feet as wide apart as your legs are long–lunge with your front leg. Lift your arms to the sky. Point your front toes straight ahead, turn in your back toes slightly.

Holding the pose

Let your lower body sink. Let your upper body lift. Straighten your elbows, and keep your fingers active (straighten them, don't let them go limp). Press the outer edge of your back leg into the floor. Square your hips and shoulders to the front. Lift your chest and move it forward. Drop your tailbone. Keep moving away from the navel center. Keep your feet in alignment. Don't move your knee past your ankle. Bring the triceps behind the ears. Switch sides. Stay an equal amount of time on each side.

WARRIOR II

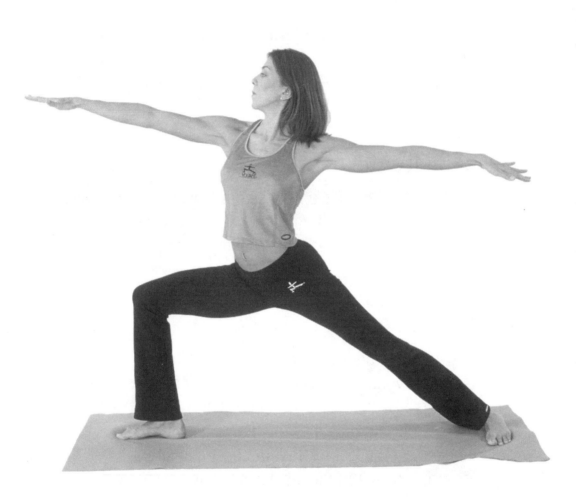

WARRIOR II

 Strengthens: Quads • Glutes
Stretches: Chest • Adductors

Warrior II typically follows Warrior I during Mountain II; it helps to improve focus and discipline.

Getting into the pose

Stand with your feet wide apart. Point your front toes straight ahead, turn in your back toes slightly. Extend your arms out at shoulder height. Bend your front knee, and keep your hips level.

Holding the pose

Focus on the front hand. Keep the fingers active. Drop your lower body, and lift your upper body. Don't let your bent knee fall inward or outward. Keep it bent at a 90-degree angle, or as close to that as possible. Tuck your tailbone. Tighten your abs. Watch your knee-to-ankle alignment (knee should not come over ankle). Switch sides.

REVERSE WARRIOR

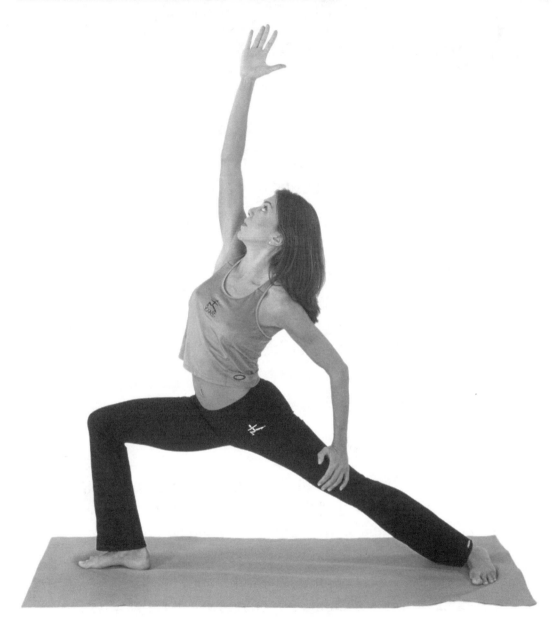

REVERSE WARRIOR

 Strengthens: Quads • Glutes
Stretches: Adductors • Waist • Lats

The Reverse Warrior follows Warrior II during Mountain II.

Getting into the pose

Stand with your feet wide apart. Point your front toes straight ahead, and turn in your back toes slightly. Bend your front knee. Lift your forward arm to the sky. Your back arm drops onto your back leg. Hips are squared to the side.

Holding the pose

Let your lower body sink. The upper body lifts. Stretch your waist and ribs. Watch your knee-to-ankle alignment. Switch sides.

TRIANGLE

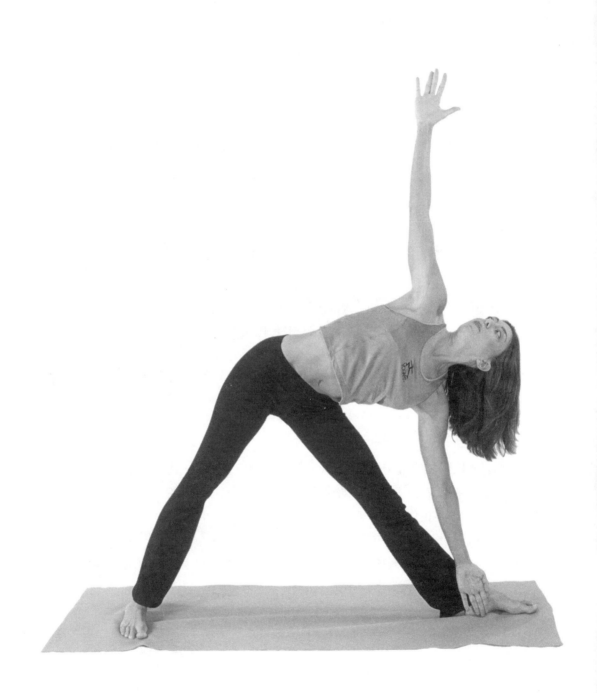

TRIANGLE

Strengthens: Torso
Stretches: Hamstrings • Waist

Use the Triangle pose during Mountain II.

Getting into the pose

Stand with your feet wide apart. Point your front toes straight ahead, and turn in your back toes slightly. Extend your arms out at shoulder height, reach your front arm forward, then drop it to your ankle or shin. Lift your back arm to the sky and open your chest. Look up to your arm, or, if your neck bothers you, look down to the floor. Your body should be flat and in line with your heels.

Holding the pose

Press your feet away from each other. Don't let your upper body fall out of alignment with your heels. Switch sides.
Advanced: Stretch your lifted arm over your ear and reach forward. Roll your upper body toward the sky.

Modification

If your hamstrings are tight, use a block.

SPINAL BALANCE

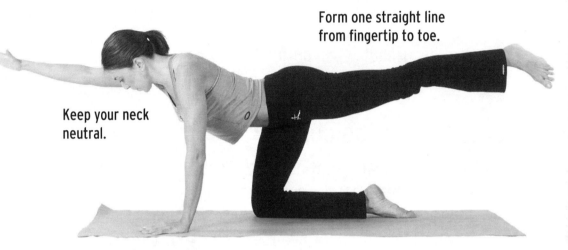

Form one straight line
from fingertip to toe.

Keep your neck
neutral.

Keep this hand
directly under
your shoulder.

SPINAL BALANCE

Strengthens: Back muscles

This one is especially helpful between poses and during warm-up, to improve balance and lengthen the spine. Use this pose during Mountain I or II.

Getting into the pose

From the hands and knees, extend one arm and the opposite leg parallel to the floor.

Holding the pose

Pull energy from the center of the body. Keep a straight spine (don't drop or lift your head). Lengthen on each exhalation. Switch sides.

Modification

Be careful if you have knee problems; use a knee pad.

TREE

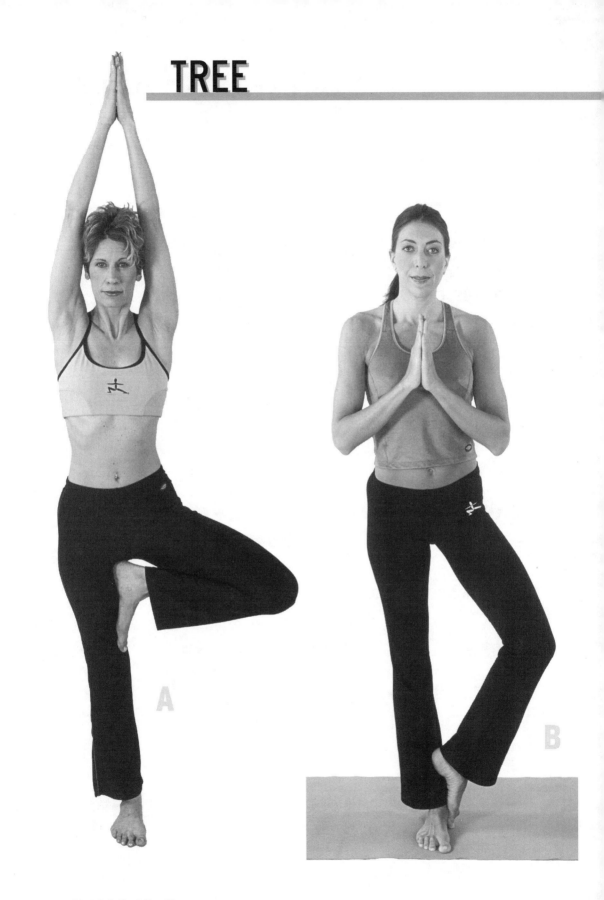

A

B

Strengthens: Quads • Glutes
Stretches: Adductors • Lats

After the body is warm, during Mountain II, assume the tree pose to promote balance and a feeling of being grounded.

Getting into the pose

Balance on one leg. Bring the opposite foot onto your standing ankle, calf, or thigh. Keep your hands in the prayer position, or for more challenge, bring your arms overhead (A).

Holding the pose

Keep drawing energy up toward the sky, and firmly root the standing foot. Contract your abs and lift out of the standing leg.

Modifications

Keep your hands in the prayer position at your heart center if you have difficulty balancing (B). People with knee problems should use caution.

EAGLE

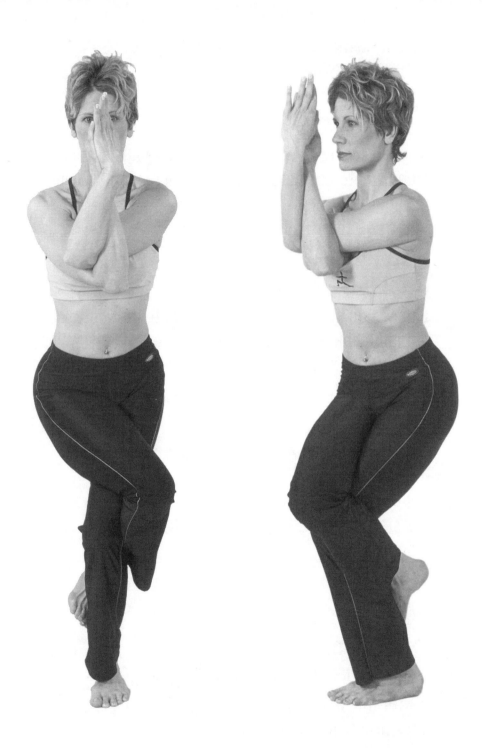

EAGLE

Strengthens: Quads • Glutes
Stretches: Hips • Rhomboids • Posterior deltoids • Calves

Similar to the Tree, this pose works well after the body is warm (during Mountain II) to improve balance and focus.

Getting into the pose

Standing on one leg, wrap the other leg around it or touch the foot to the floor. Squat and cross the same side arm as your top leg under the other. Touch hands (or palms) together if possible.

Holding the pose

Keep drawing energy up toward the sky, and firmly root the standing foot. Contract your abs; keep your tailbone low.

Modification

People with knee problems should use caution.

BALANCING HALF-MOON

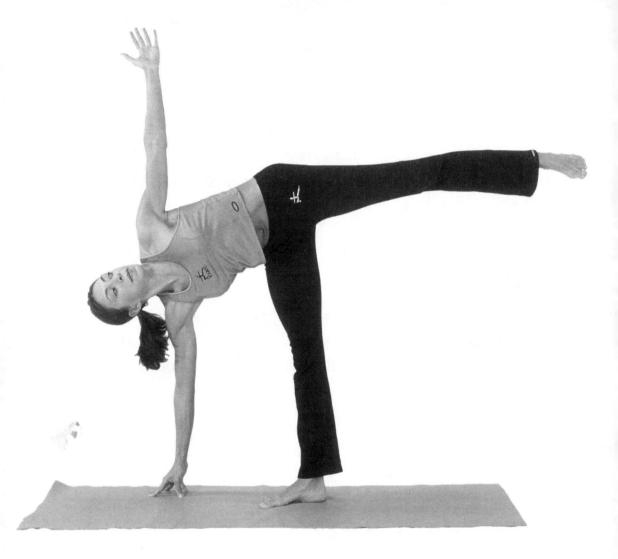

BALANCING HALF-MOON

 Strengthens: Obliques • Adductors
Stretches: Hamstrings

As its title suggests, this pose is another balance improver. Use only after the body is *thoroughly* warm, during Mountain II.

Getting into the pose

From a wide stance, raise your back leg to the height of your hip. Bring your back hand to your hip, with your front fingertips on the floor, directly under the front shoulder.

Holding the pose

If comfortable, reach your top arm to the sky. Stay focused. If balanced, look up to the top hand. Switch sides.

Modifications

If your hamstrings are tight, use a block. People with shoulder instability and rotator cuff injuries may want to avoid this pose.

EXTENDED ANGLE

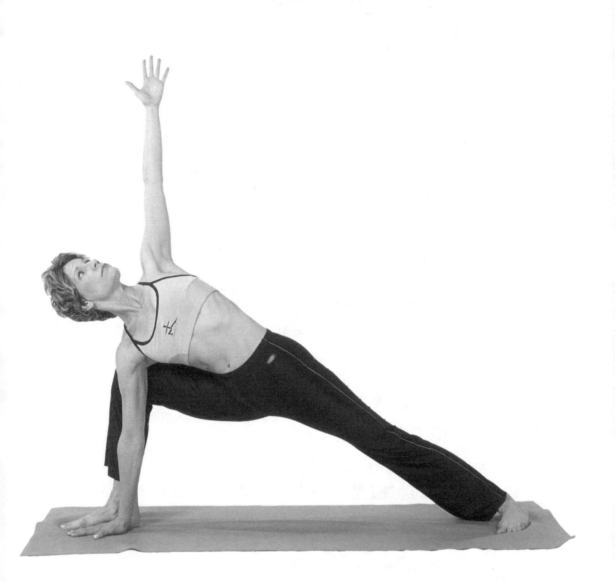

EXTENDED ANGLE

Strengthens: Quads
Stretches: Groin • Waist

Use this pose during Mountain II.

Getting into the pose

Stand with your feet wide apart. Point your front toes straight ahead, and turn in your back toes slightly. Bend your front knee, bring your front arm down, with hand inside the front foot, lining your arm up with your lower leg; extend your top arm to the sky. If comfortable, look up.

Holding the pose

Rotate your chest up to the sky; press your hand into the ground. Press your elbow into your knee. Sink into your bent knee. Tighten the glutes and push your hips forward as you extend the line of energy from the tailbone to the crown of the head. Switch sides.

SUN GOD

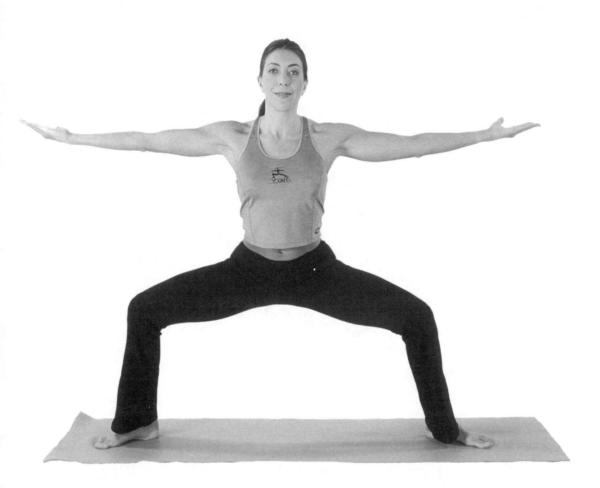

SUN GOD

Strengthens: Glutes • Quads • Adductors

This pose is used during Mountain II. It strengthens and tones your legs.

Getting into the pose

Come to a wide stance (sideways on your mat), with your feet turned out. Extend your arms out at shoulder height, palms facing up. Slowly sink your hips and then hold. Squeeze your inner thighs to come back up.

Holding the pose

Make sure your weight is on your heels and your spine is straight.

BOAT

BOAT

Strengthens: Abs • Hip flexors • Quads

The Boat is used after the Seated Forward Fold (pages 62-63), when the body is warm during Mountain III. It fosters a centered feeling and improves balance.

Getting into the pose

From the Seated Forward Fold, lift your legs and arms. Stay on sitting bones.

Holding the pose

Bring heat, strength, and energy from the center of your body outward to your legs and arms. Focus on the breath. Balance on your sitting bones, and lift your ribcage.

Modification

If you have back injuries or are a beginner, bend your knees and hold the backs of your thighs or knees.

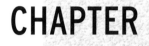

4

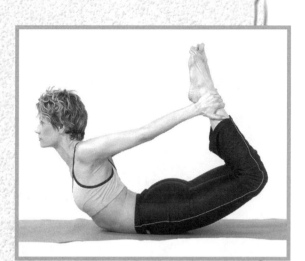

Forward Bends and Back Bends

STANDING CHEST EXPANSION

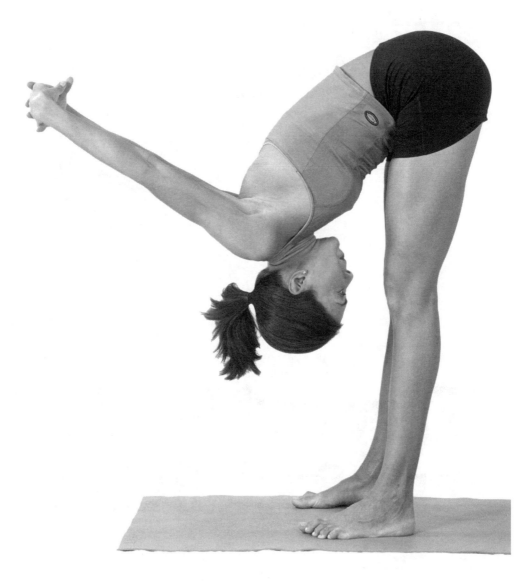

STANDING CHEST EXPANSION

 Stretches: Hamstrings • Deltoids • Pectorals

Use this pose before, during, and after any upper body work, to stretch shoulders and chest, during Mountain I, II, or III.

Getting into the pose

Interlace your hands behind your back. Lift your arms up toward your upper back. Lift your chest, then lead with the chest into a forward fold, with your knees slightly bent.

Holding the pose

Breathe into your shoulders. Lift your tailbone to the sky. Drop your head, neck, and chest toward the floor. Let the breath take you into your body. Tighten your abdominal muscles.

Modifications

Use straps or a towel when your shoulders are tight.

Bend your knees to protect your lower back.

People with disc injuries should not attempt this pose.

MONKEY AND
WRIST STRETCH

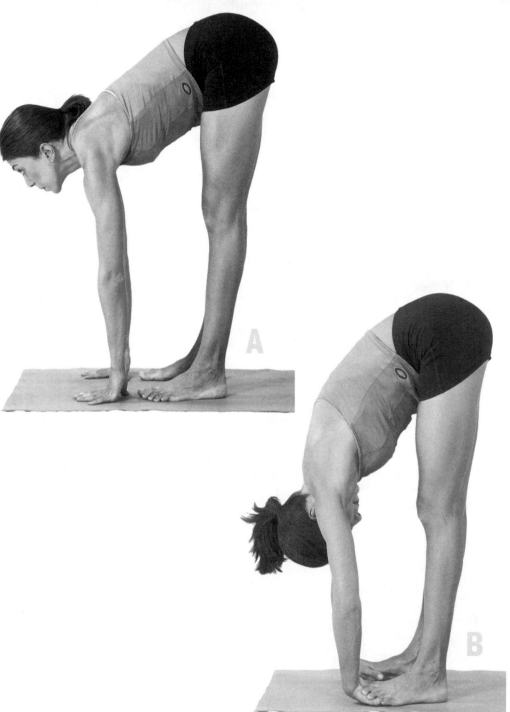

MONKEY AND WRIST STRETCH

Strengthens: Back
Stretches: Hamstrings

These stretches are effective to use before, after, and between Downward Facing Dog (pages 66-67), and during Mountain I or II. The position lengthens the neck and relieves carpal tunnel syndrome.

Getting into the pose

Monkey Stretch (A): Place your feet slightly apart (up to hip width). Fold your upper body forward and down. Place your fingertips on the floor in front of your feet. Inhale and lift your chest away from your thighs. Look up, and straighten your back. Exhale and forward fold again.

Wrist Stretch (B): Same as the Monkey, only bend your knees and slide your hands underneath your feet until your toes touch the inside of your wrists.

Holding the pose

Monkey Stretch: Hold your head up; keep your back flat.

Wrist Stretch: Slowly attempt to straighten your legs as much as possible and comfortable.

Modifications

Students with lower back problems, sciatica, or tight hamstrings should bend their knees. People with sciatica should always bend their knees in forward folds. If you cannot reach the ground or have disc problems, keep your hands on your thighs.

STANDING FORWARD FOLD

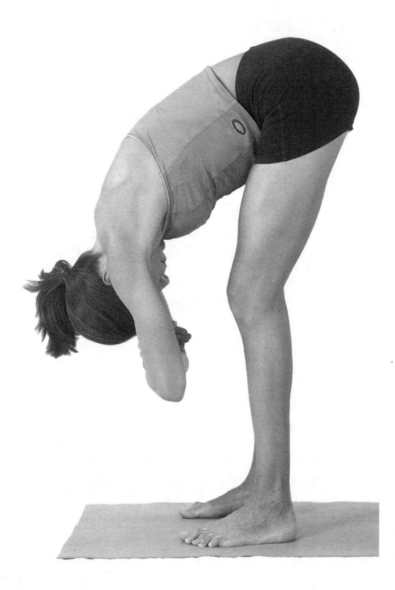

STANDING FORWARD FOLD

 Stretches: Hamstrings • Back

Use the Standing Forward Fold as a transition during Mountain I or II.

Getting into the pose

Place your feet hip-width apart. Lift your arms to the sky. Extend your arms out and bring them down in front of your feet, if you can. Keep your knees bent to protect your lower back. Grab your elbows if you like, then rest your hands inside your elbow creases.

Holding the pose

Lift your tailbone to the sky. Relax your head and neck (shake out your head; sigh). Breathe into the lower back and hamstrings. Tighten your abs.

Modification

Keep your knees bent if you have back problems, sciatica, or tight hamstrings.

AIRPLANE

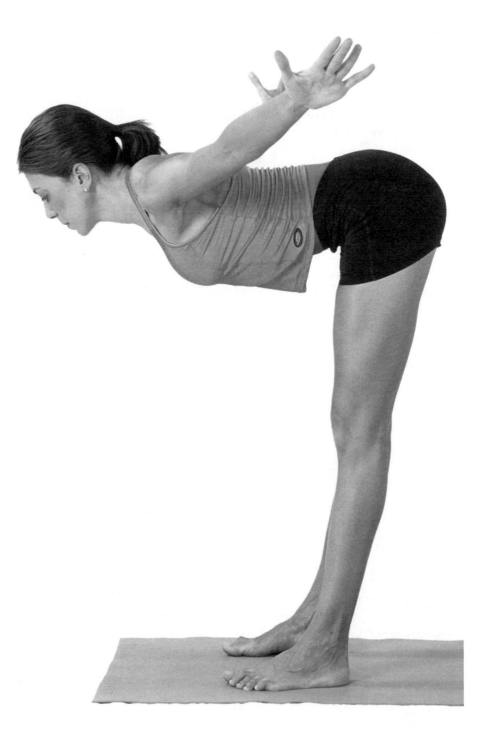

AIRPLANE

 Strengthens: Back muscles
Stretches: Hamstrings

During transitions between back and forward bends, get into the Airplane pose to elongate the spine. Use during Mountain I or II.

Getting into the pose

Standing, lift your arms over your head. Spread your arms out to shoulder height and draw them back. Hinge forward half way and draw your shoulder blades together.

Holding the pose

Pull energy from your chest to your fingertips. Look down at the floor. Visualize a light or energy moving from your tailbone through the top of your head. Keep your back flat. Draw your back muscles together, and lift your arms high. Your palms should face the floor.

Modification

Bend your knees if you have lower back problems, sciatica, or tight hamstrings.

PYRAMID

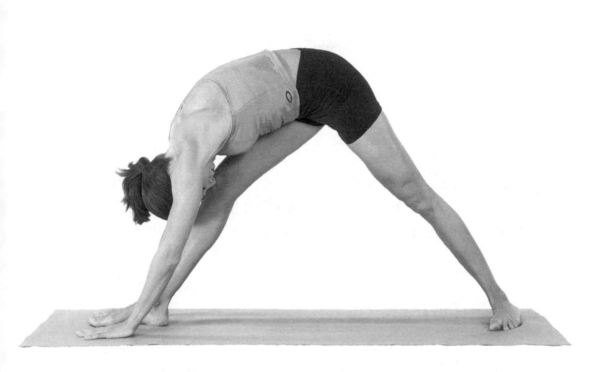

PYRAMID

Stretches: Hamstrings • Lower back • Hips

The Pyramid is used often out of Warrior I, or before Reverse Twisting Triangle (pages 86-87), during Mountain II or III.

Getting into the pose

Stand with your feet wide apart. Point your front toes straight ahead, with your back toes turned in slightly. Lower down over your front leg. Move your head to your knee.

Holding the pose

Bend your knee until your head meets your knee, then, keeping your head and knee together, straighten your leg. Bend and straighten your legs a few times. Keep your knee bent if your forehead does not reach the knee otherwise. Don't hyperextend the knees. Relax the head and neck. Switch sides.

Modifications

Bend the front knee. Use a block if you have tight hamstrings.

STANDING STRADDLE SPLITS

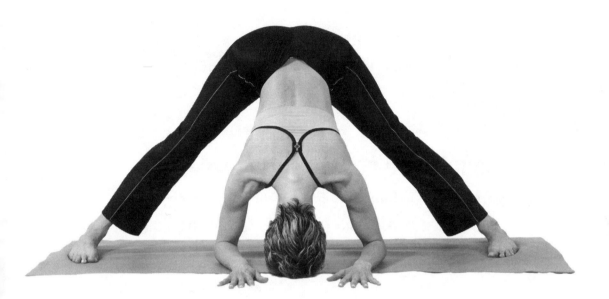

STANDING STRADDLE SPLITS

Stretches: Groin • Inner thighs • Hamstrings

Use this pose when the hamstrings are warm, during Mountain II or III.

Getting into the pose

Stand with your feet wide apart, toes facing forward. Place your palms flat on the floor, if possible. Push your feet out.

Holding the pose

Bring your elbows down to the floor. If possible, bring the top of your head to the floor.

Modification

People with groin injuries should avoid this pose.

SEATED FORWARD FOLD

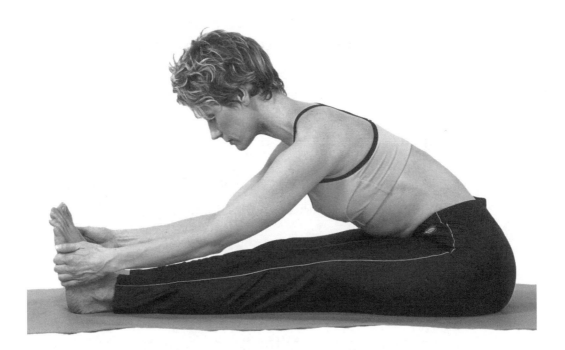

SEATED FORWARD FOLD

 Stretches: Hamstrings • Lower back

Use the Seated Forward Fold only after the body is *thoroughly* warm, during Mountain III.

Getting into the pose

From a seated position, extend your legs. Pull your toes back toward your body. Lift your arms. Hinge at the hips and fall forward.

Holding the pose

Let your hands rest on your legs, knees, ankles, feet, or the floor. Relax your shoulders.

Advanced: Grab hold of your feet wherever you can (sides, toes, heels), and push your upper body forward. Don't force this stretch. Breathe into your lower back. It does not matter whether you can reach your toes or only your knees.

Modifications

Use straps or a towel if your hamstrings are tight.
Bend your knees if necessary.

SEATED STRADDLE SPLITS

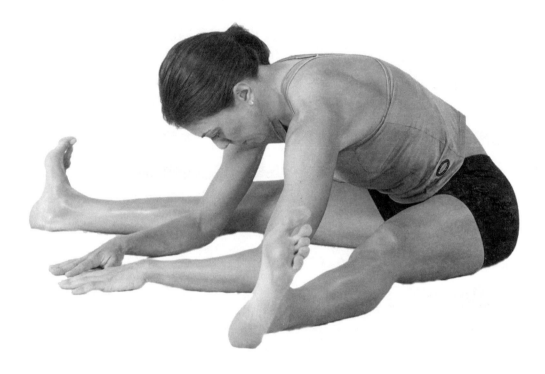

SEATED STRADDLE SPLITS

Stretches: Hamstrings • Lower back

Use the Seated Straddle Splits after the body is warm, during Mountain III.

Getting into the pose

From a seated position, separate the legs out wide. Hinge at your hips and fall forward. Bend your knees if necessary.

Holding the pose

Breathe into your back. Pull your toes back toward your body. Tighten your midsection.

Modification
Bend your knees.

DOWNWARD FACING DOG

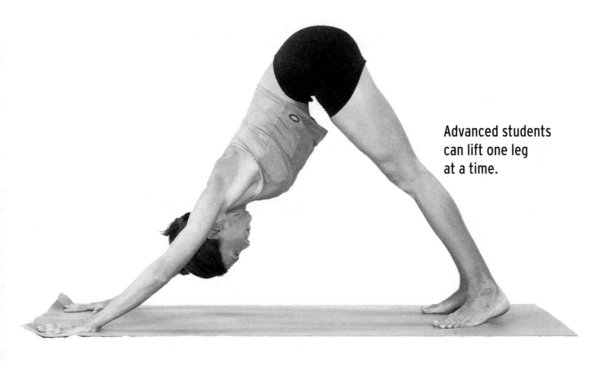

Advanced students
can lift one leg
at a time.

DOWNWARD FACING DOG

 Strengthens: Upper body
Stretches: Shoulders • Hamstrings

The Downward Facing Dog pose is great to use after warm-up as a transition between many poses, during Mountains I and II.

Getting into the pose

Place your palms flat on the floor, shoulder width apart, fingers fanned out. Step back and press your feet into the floor.

Holding the pose

Lift your tailbone to the sky. Push your palms forward and heels back. Let your chest, head, and neck sink into the floor. Breathe into the back.

Modifications

Drop your knees.

CAT-COW STRETCH

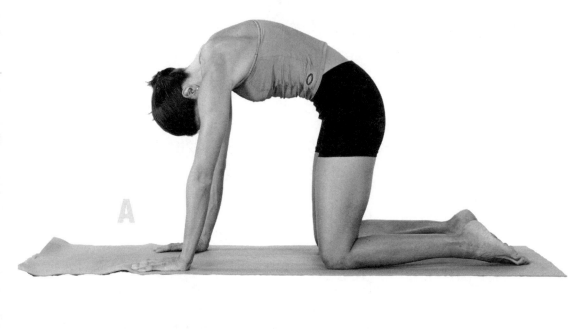

A

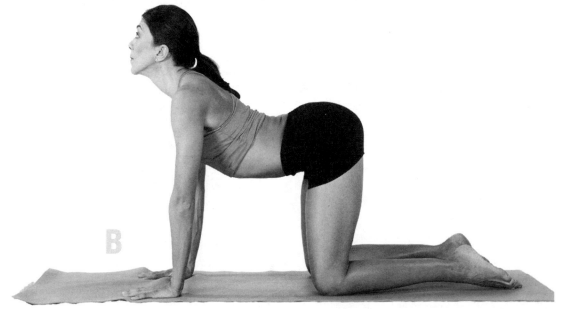

B

CAT–COW STRETCH

 Strengthens: Abdominals • Neck • Front and back of torso
Stretches: Abdominals • Torso

Use this pose to warm up the torso, often during
Mountain I.

Getting into the pose

Start from your hands and knees. First, round your back
up to the sky (A), then arch your back with your head
up (B).

Holding the pose

Move with the breath. Alternate cat (rounding) with cow
(arching). Inhale up (cow) and exhale down (cat).

STANDING BACK BEND

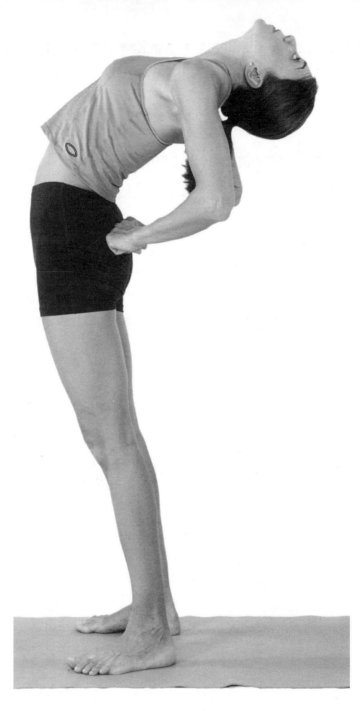

STANDING BACK BEND

 Strengthens: Glutes • Back • Abdominals
Stretches: Front of body

Back bends are great for slowing the aging process and relieving stress. Make sure to use it only when warm, especially during Mountain II. Always follow back bends with forward bends.

Getting into the pose

Place your hands or fists on your upper hips. Push forward through the midsection. Lift your chest to the sky.

Holding the pose

Keep lifting out of your lower back. If comfortable, drop your head and neck back. Keep lifting your chest to the sky. Keep the glutes tight. Draw the quads up.

Modification

Back bends may aggravate lower back problems, so use caution.

SUNBIRD

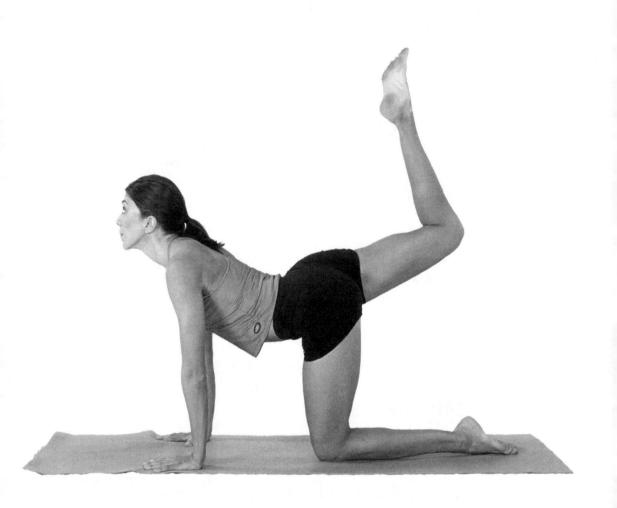

SUNBIRD

 Strengthens and stretches: Back of the body • Front of the body

Use the Sunbird pose during Mountain I or II.

Getting into the pose

From your hands and knees, exhale and bring one knee under the body, toward the forehead. Then inhale and extend that same leg back and up to the sky. Contract your abs.

Holding the pose

Move energy from the center of your body. Keep the back of your neck long. Switch sides.

Modification

If you have sensitive knees or knee problems, use extra padding.

CAMEL

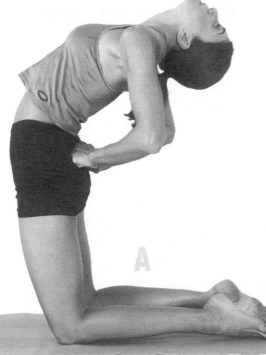

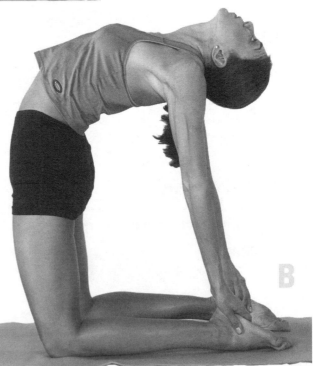

Strengthens: Back of body
Stretches: Front of body • Quads

Use the Camel after Standing Back Bend (pages 70-71), during Mountain III.

Getting into the pose

Move slowly. From a kneeling position, lift your arms and place your hands on your hips (A). Push your hips forward. Lift your chest to the sky. Relax your head, neck, and back.

Holding the pose

Keep lifting out of your lower back and pushing your hips forward. Keep your glutes very tight to protect your lower back.

Modifications

Use extra padding for your knees in case of knee problems or sensitivities.

Advanced: Drop your arms behind you, and grab onto your heels (toes under, or, more challenging, feet flat). See photo B.

SUPERMAN

Look forward, and avoid
overstretching your neck.

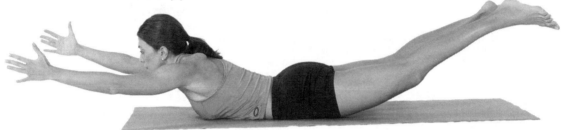

Lift arms, chest, and
legs off the ground.

SUPERMAN

 Strengthens: Back of body
Stretches: Front of body

The Superman pose strengthens the back muscles; use it during Mountain II or III.

Getting into the pose

Lie down on your stomach. Extend your arms forward with your legs straight back. Lift your arms and legs.

Holding the pose

Lift and pull your limbs away from your torso.

Modification

Bring your arms down to your sides.

BOW

Strengthens: Back of body
Stretches: Front of body

The Bow pose stretches the front of the body and is typically used during Mountain III.

Getting into the pose

Lying on your stomach, reach back and grab your right ankle with your right hand and your left ankle with your left hand. Extend your chest and legs to the sky. Pull your ankles back.

Holding the pose

Keep breathing into your chest. Lift out of your lower back. Push your legs together. Pull your arms and legs to the sky.

Modification

If you can't reach your ankles with your hands, use straps.

COBRA

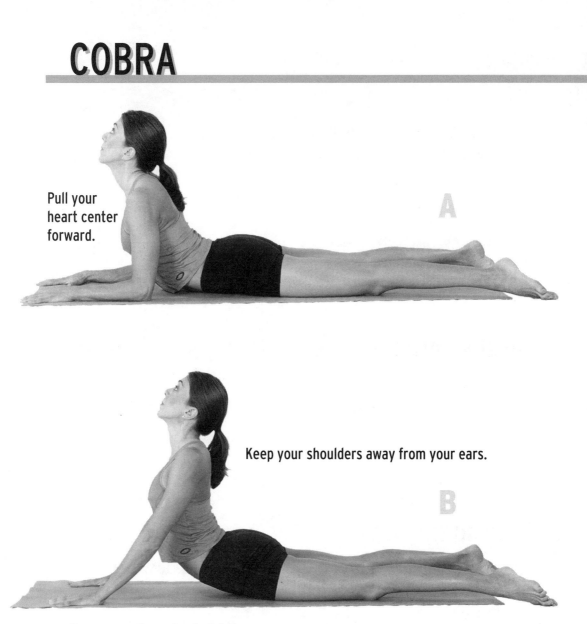

Pull your heart center forward.

A

Keep your shoulders away from your ears.

B

Keep your elbows bent slightly.

COBRA

Strengthens: Arms • Shoulders • Back
Stretches: Chest • Abdominals

The Cobra is a chest opener. Use only when your back is warm.

Getting into the pose

Lying on your stomach, bring your elbows under your shoulders (hands forward). Stretch your chest to the sky (A).

Holding the pose

Advanced: Push your palms into the floor and pull your chest higher (B). The hips should stay on the ground.

BRIDGE

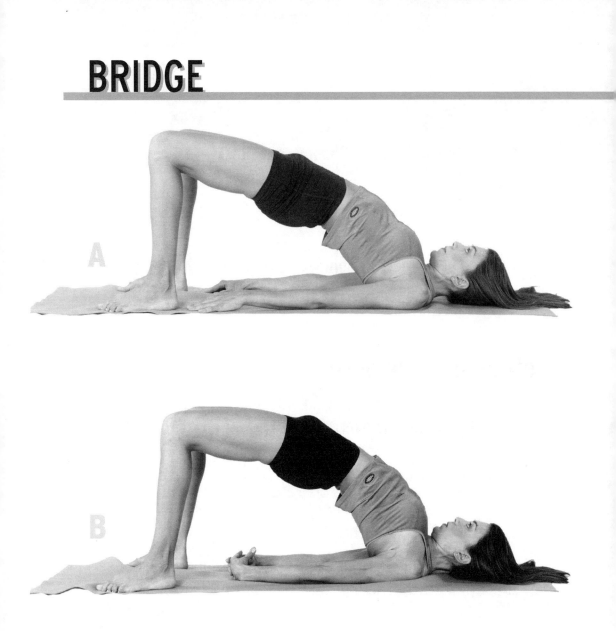

BRIDGE

 Strengthens: Glutes • Hamstrings • Calves
Stretches: Abdominals • Chest

Assume this pose to open the front of your body and
stretch your midsection.

Getting into the pose

Lie down on your back, with your palms facedown. Bring
the soles of your feet to the floor (knees up), hip-width
apart. Lift your hips to the sky. Push your hips up and your
heels into the ground (A).

Holding the pose

Advanced: Interlace your hands under your body (B). Bring
your shoulders under so your body is resting on the outside edge of your shoulders. Breathe into the navel center.

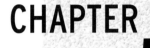

5

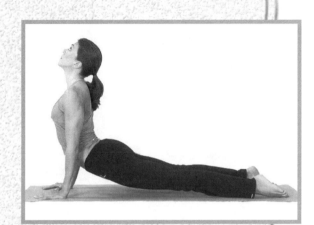

Twists, Planks, and Ab Work

REVERSE TWISTING TRIANGLE

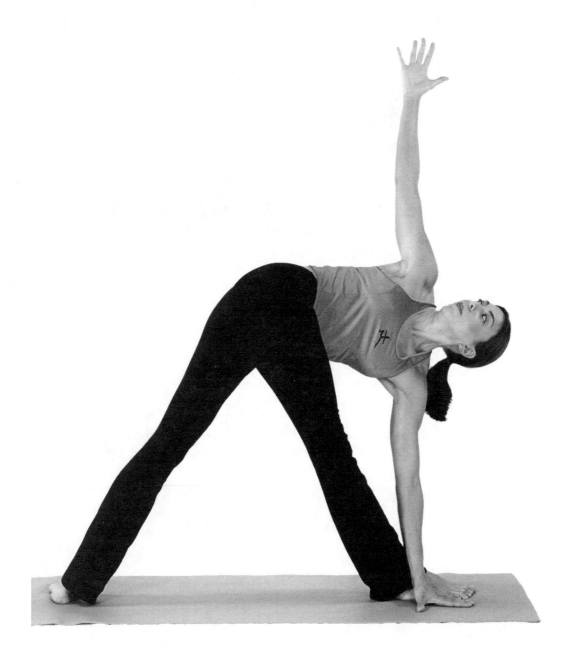

REVERSE TWISTING TRIANGLE

Strengthens: Obliques • Waist
Stretches: Hips • Hamstrings

Twisting poses stimulate the internal organs. Use this pose during Mountain II, typically after the Pyramid or Triangle.

Getting into the pose

Stand with your feet wide apart. Point your front toes straight ahead, with your back toes turned in slightly. Bring your left hand to your right ankle or the floor. Move your right arm up to the sky.

Holding the pose

Your feet should be close enough together that the legs are able to straighten. Open your chest to the sky. Breathe into your waist. Look up to the right hand. Switch sides.

Modification

If you have tight hamstrings, use a block.

Caution: The rotation/flexion in this pose may aggravate a disc injury.

LYING DOWN SPINAL TWIST

Try to keep both
shoulders on the floor.

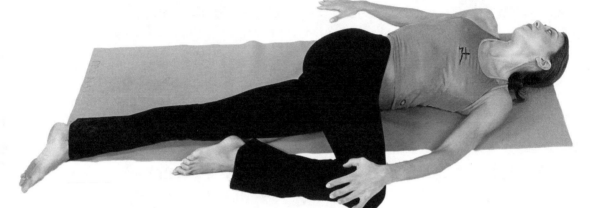

Use your hand to help move your
knee toward the floor (gently!).

LYING DOWN SPINAL TWIST

 Stretches: Lower back • Torso • Hips • Shoulders

Use this position to release your lower back after standing postures. It also stimulates the internal organs.

Getting into the pose

Lie down on the floor. Bring your right knee into your chest. Extend your left leg to the floor. Bring your right knee to the left side of your body.

Holding the pose

Place your left hand on your right leg, gently pressing it downward. Look over your right shoulder. Try to keep both shoulders on the ground. Breathe into the body. Switch sides.

SEATED TWIST

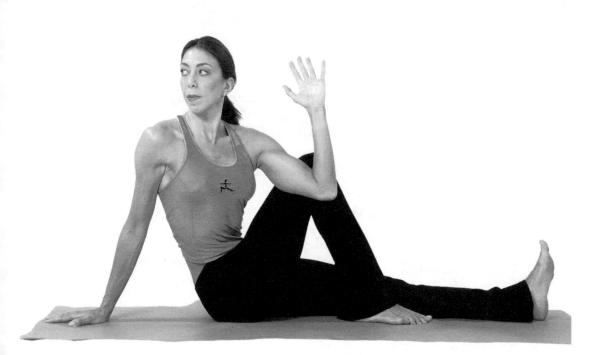

SEATED TWIST

Stretches: Waist • Midsection • Spine

After your spine is warm, use this pose to release your upper back. It is also beneficial in stimulating the internal organs.

Getting into the pose

From a seated position, extend your legs out. Bring your right knee up with the sole of your foot on the floor. Place your left elbow outside your right knee, and twist your body at the waist.

Holding the pose

Use the breath. Twist further on every exhalation.

PLANK

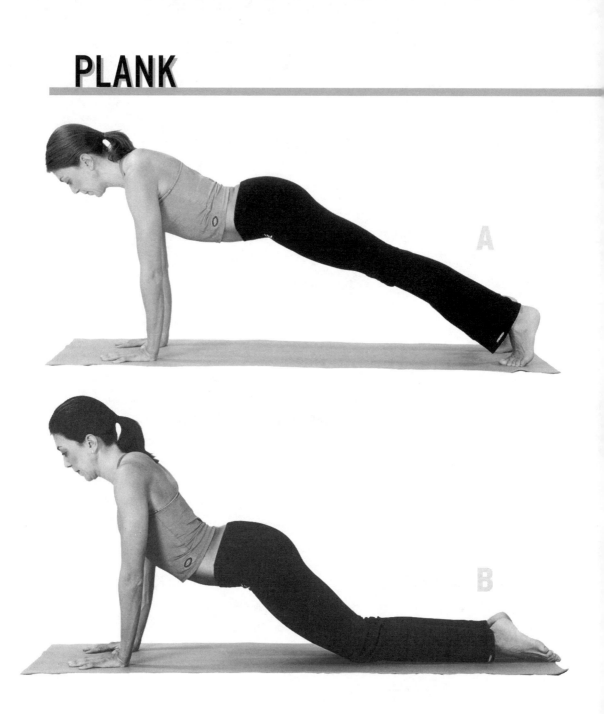

A

B

PLANK

Strengthens: Arms • Shoulders • Chest • Abdominals

The Plank is used to work the upper body, during Mountains I and II.

Getting into the pose

From Downward Facing Dog, move forward until your shoulders are over your hands (A). Keep your back straight, like a plank, and your midsection strong.

Holding the pose

Keep your body aligned, hips slightly elevated.

Modification

Beginners: Drop your knees (B).

CROCODILE

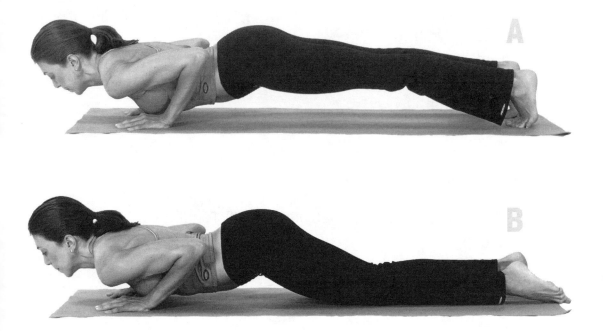

A

B

CROCODILE

Strengthens: Arms • Shoulders • Chest • Abdominals

Use the Crocodile to work the upper body during Mountains I and II.

Getting into the pose

From the Plank, lower your chest down while your elbows are tucked in and "hug" your ribcage. Your hands are directly under your shoulders, your hips are elevated slightly (A).

Holding the pose

Keep the body aligned. Move slowly.

Modification

Beginners: Drop your knees (B).

UPWARD FACING DOG

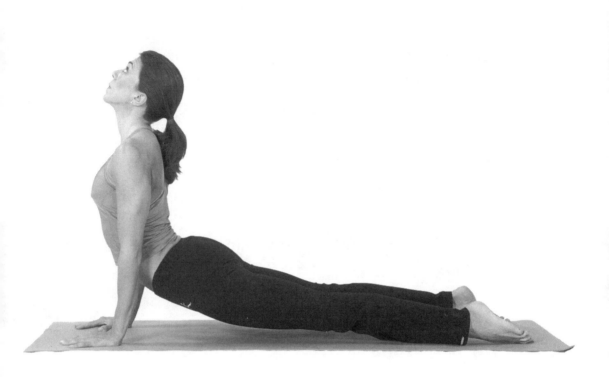

UPWARD FACING DOG

 Strengthens: Shoulders • Arms • Quads • Lats
Stretches: Front of body

Use this pose after Downward Facing Dog and Crocodile, to stretch the front of your body. Use it during Mountains I and II.

Getting into the pose

From Crocodile, pull your upper body forward and up. Arch your back and bring your chest to the sky. Be sure to "pull," not to push up.

Holding the pose

Keep your elbows unlocked and your shoulders away from your ears. Keep your leg muscles and glutes tight to protect your lower back. Tighten the back of your body.

Modifications

Beginners: Drop your knees.

INCLINE PLANK

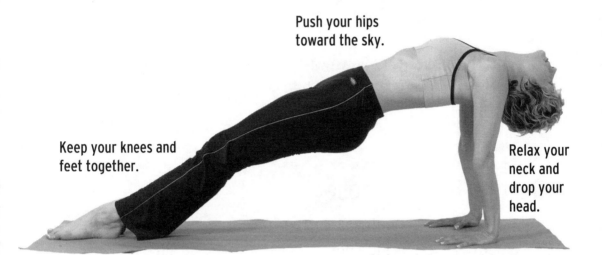

Push your hips toward the sky.

Keep your knees and feet together.

Relax your neck and drop your head.

INCLINE PLANK

Strengthens: Glutes • Arms
Stretches: Front of body

Use the Incline Plank after or before a Seated Forward Fold, during Mountain II or III.

Getting into the pose

From a seated position, extend your legs. Place your palms on the floor behind you with your fingers spread and pointing toward your body. Press your hips up and get your body as straight as a plank, using your hands and feet.

Holding the pose

Keep your arms straight. Pull your toes out and down. Relax your neck.

Modification

Make fists to protect your wrists.

TABLETOP

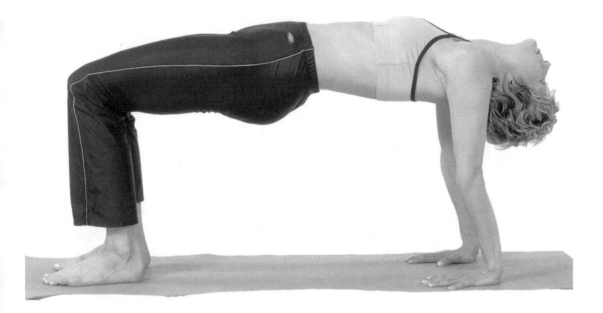

TABLETOP

Strengthens: Glutes • Arms
Stretches: Front of body

Use the this pose instead of or in combination with the Incline Plank, during Mountain II or III.

Getting into the pose

From a seated position, extend your legs. Place your palms on the floor behind you with your fingers spread and pointing toward your body. Put the soles of your feet on the floor, about hip-width apart. Press your hips up and keep your knees bent. Press into your palms and feet.

Holding the pose

Push your hips up. Relax your neck back or look up.

Modification

Make fists to protect your wrists.

KNEELING SIDE PLANK

A

B

KNEELING SIDE PLANK

 Strengthens: Obliques • Shoulders • Intercostals
Stretches: Obliques • Intercostals

Use this plank pose during Mountain I or II.

Getting into the pose

From the Plank, drop your left knee. With your left hand on the floor, raise your right arm and open the right side of the body (A). Your right leg is straight with the inside edge of your right foot on the floor.

Holding the pose

Open the right side of your chest to the sky. Pull energy from the navel center up to the hands. Switch sides.

Modifications

Use extra padding for your knees in case of knee problems or sensitivities.

Advanced: Straighten out both legs and balance on the outside edge of your left foot and the inside edge of your right foot (B). This version is called Side Plank.

AB WORK

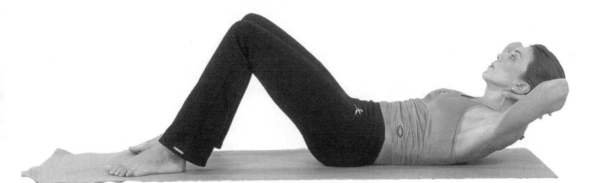

A

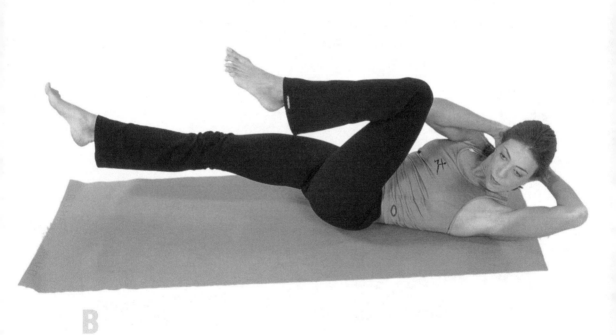

B

AB WORK

Strengthens: Abdominals • Obliques • Hip flexors

Besides strengthening the abs, this stretch fosters a feeling of being centered, strengthens your power center (midsection), and enhances self-esteem. Use it during Mountain II or III.

Getting into the pose

Start with your back on the floor and your knees up (your feet are on the floor). Place your hands behind your head with the fingers interlaced (thumbs along neck) to support your head. Your elbows are out to your sides. Slowly lift your head, neck, and shoulders on an exhalation (A). Look straight up. Hold, and then move down slowly on the inhalation.

Holding the pose

Press your lower back into the ground. Do not protrude your stomach on the exhale. Keep the elbows wide. For oblique work, bring your knee to your chest and twist one shoulder to the opposite knee (B).

6

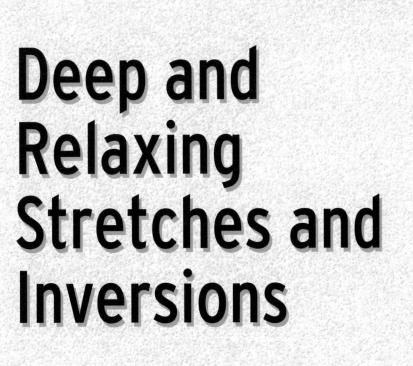

Deep and Relaxing Stretches and Inversions

CHILD'S POSE

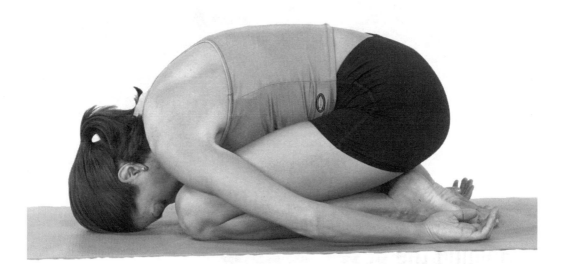

CHILD'S POSE

Stretches: Back muscles

Between poses, rest and check in with your body in the Child's Pose.

Getting into the pose

From your hands and knees, push back and bring your arms around to the sides of your body.

Holding the pose

Rest and breathe. Check in with your body.

Modification

Extend your arms out in front of you. This modification is called Extended Child's Pose.

FROG

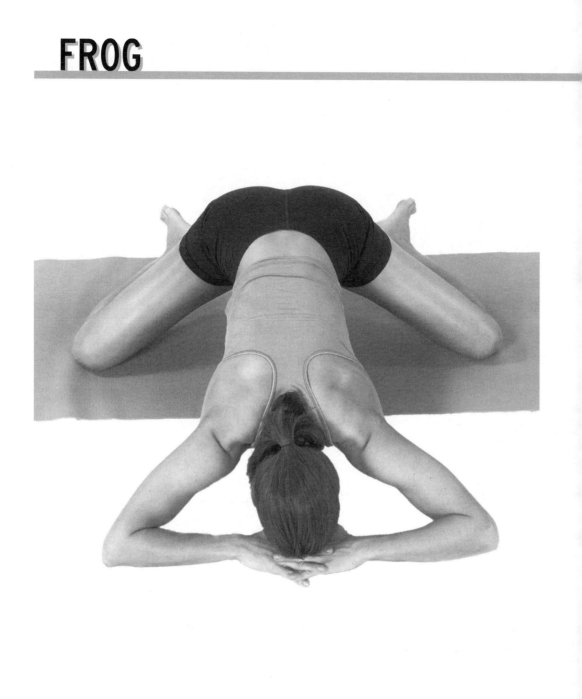

Stretches: Groin

This pose provides rest and relaxation. Use after your body is warm, during Mountain III.

Getting into the pose

Kneel on the floor. Separate your knees widely out to the sides. Bring your upper body down toward the floor.

Holding the pose

Keep pushing your hips back. Lower your chest to the floor. Keep your spine neutral. Keep your abs firm.

Modification

Avoid this pose if you have knee injuries.

KNOT

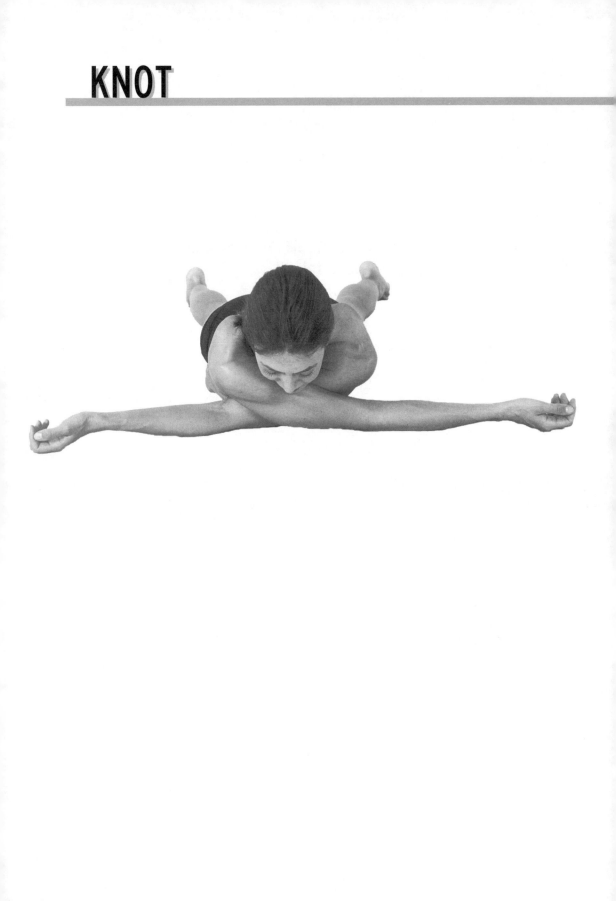

KNOT

Stretches: Shoulders • Deltoids • Rhomboids

Stretch your shoulders and deltoids with the Knot pose. Weightlifters will find this pose helpful in releasing the muscles after lifting. Use during Mountain III.

Getting into the pose

Lie down on your stomach. Bring one arm across your chest and the other in the opposite direction.

Holding the pose

Keep pulling your arms across each other to increase the stretch. Curl your toes, and inch your body forward over the crossed arms.

PIGEON

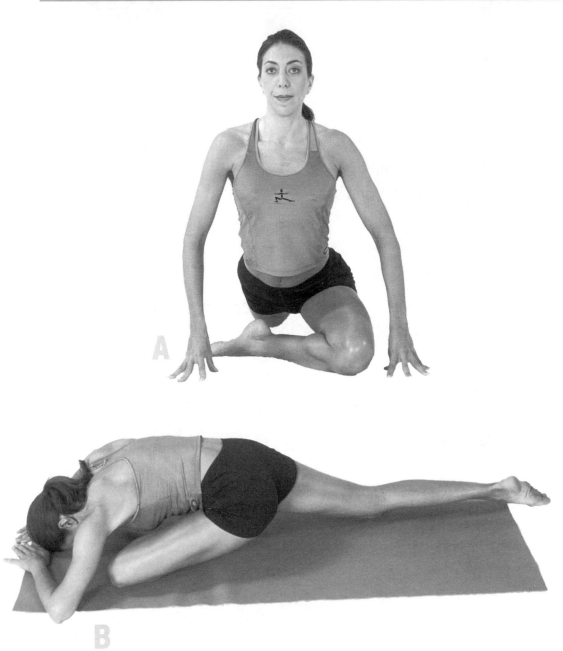

A

B

PIGEON

Stretches: Hip abductors

Use the Pigeon to stretch your hips and release stress, during Mountain II or III.

Getting into the pose

From Downward Facing Dog, lift one leg, and bring the leg forward under your body (A). Slowly lower your body down over your bent leg (B). Inhale chest up and then sink chest to the floor. Bring your arms forward.

Holding the pose

Your body should be straight and not twisted. Relax into the pose. For more intensity, bring the bent leg's foot further away from your groin. Switch sides.

Modification

If you have knee problems, be very cautious and bring your foot closer to the groin or avoid the pose completely.

PLOUGH

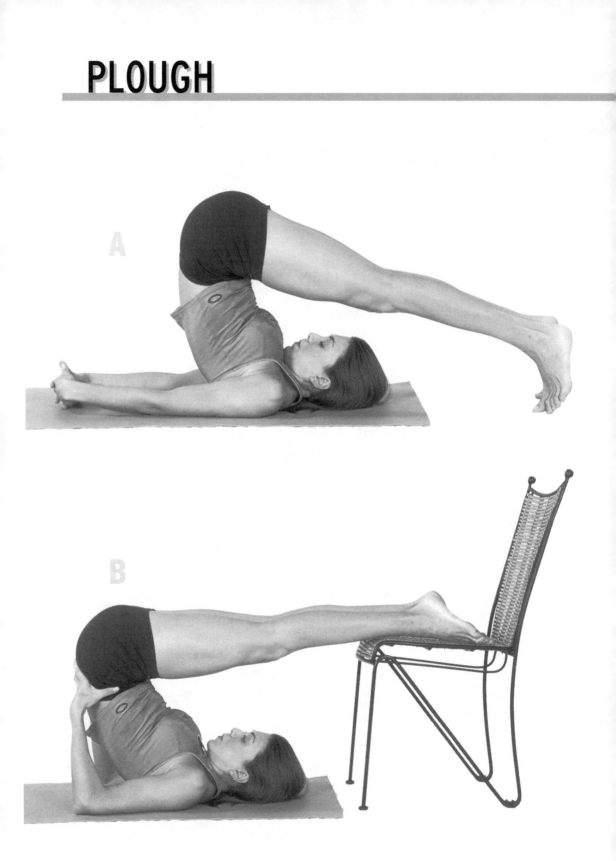

PLOUGH

Strengthens: Abdominals
Stretches: Back

The Plough is most effective near the end of class, when the body is warm. It stimulates the thyroid and increases metabolism. Use it during Mountain III.

Getting into the pose

Lying on your back, bring your legs over your head (A). Support your lower back with your hands. Straighten your legs if you can. Curl your toes.

Holding the pose

Keep your legs straight. If your feet don't touch the floor, support your lower back with your hands. Breathe easily into your throat.

Modifications

To ease pressure on your neck, roll up a towel or shirt and place it under the shoulders for support. People with neck injuries should not attempt this pose. If you cannot easily reach the floor with your feet, you can use a chair as a prop to put your legs on (B).

SHOULDER STAND

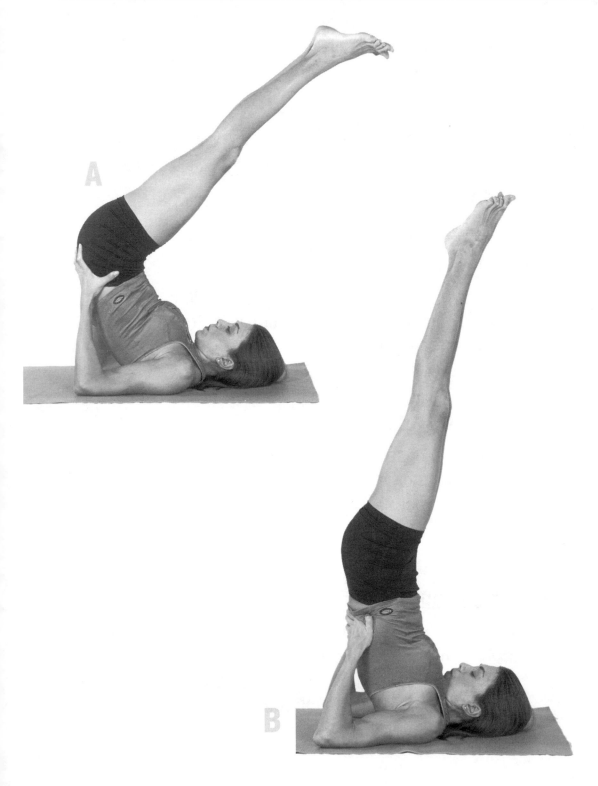

SHOULDER STAND

 Strengthens: Abdominals • Back

Use this pose after the Plough. Its many benefits include stimulating the thyroid, increasing metabolism, stimulating the internal organs, relieving varicose veins, helping reduce blood pressure, and controlling edema. It should be used during Mountain III.

Getting into the pose

Lie on your back. Lift your legs to the sky. Support your lower back with your hands (A). Don't move your neck in this pose.

Holding the pose

Use your stomach muscles and glutes to lift higher. Walk your hands up your back and move your elbows closer together. Only advanced students should attempt the fully perpendicular form of the pose (B). For less pressure on the back, bend slightly at the waist.

Modification

People who are unable to do this pose and women who are menstruating should lie on their backs and bring their legs up against a wall.

KNEES TO CHEST

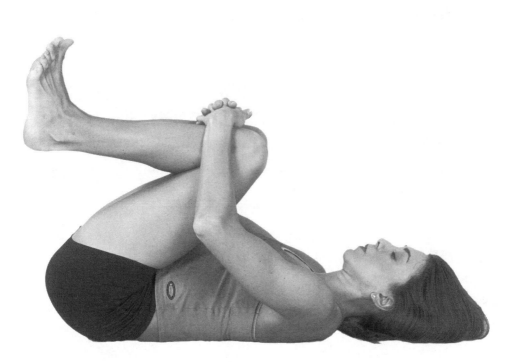

KNEES TO CHEST

Stretches: Lower back

Following back bends, release the lower back with this pose.

Getting into the pose

Lie down with your back on the floor. Bring your knees into your chest. Grab your legs under or over the knees.

Holding the pose

Keep pulling your knees toward your chest and pushing your tailbone down to the floor. For a gentle back massage, rock gently from side to side.

FISH

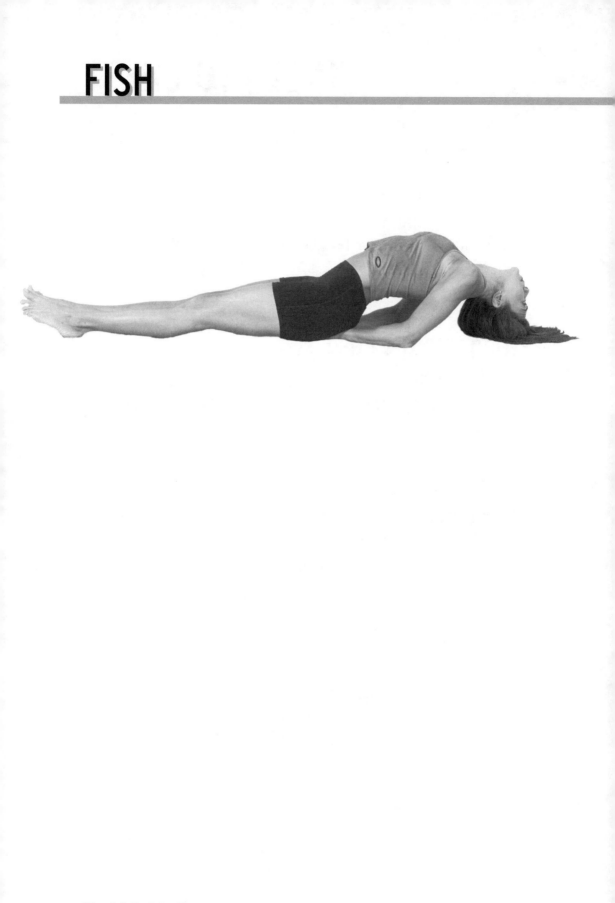

FISH

Strengthens: Rhomboids
Stretches: Chest

Assume the Fish directly after the Plough or Shoulder Stand. This pose can relieve asthma, bronchial disorders, and chest congestion. It also stimulates the thyroid and the metabolism and is a counterpose for an inversion. Use it during Mountain III.

Getting into the pose

From the Plough, bring your knees to your chest, and then lower your legs to the floor. Bring your palms under your hips and move your elbows under your body.

Holding the pose

Arch your back while your head remains on or close to the floor. Relax your head and neck.

Modification

Use a bolster under your back.

BUTTERFLY

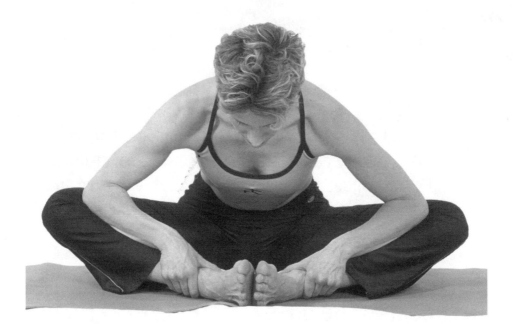

BUTTERFLY

Stretches: Hips • Lower back • Groin

Use the Butterfly after your body is warm, during Mountain III.

Getting into the pose

From a seated position, lift your chest toward the sky. Bring the soles of your feet together. Release your knees to the floor. Fold forward, holding on to your ankles.

Holding the pose

Visualize your knees sinking closer to the floor. Use your elbows to gently press the knees open.

Modification

Use caution if you have knee problems.

QUAD STRETCH

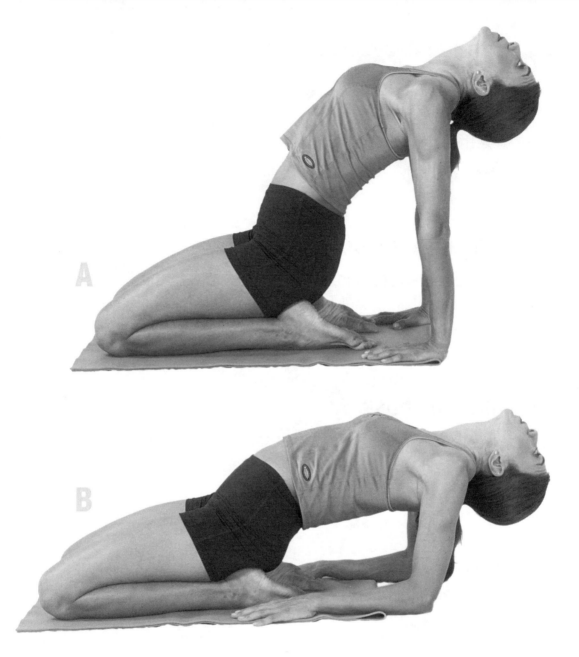

QUAD STRETCH

Strengthens: Glutes
Stretches: Quads

Use the Quad Stretch during Mountain III.

Getting into the pose

From a kneeling position, sit back on your heels. Place your hands on the floor by your hips. Arch your chest to the sky (A).

Holding the pose

Push your hips forward; lift your chest.
Advanced: Move your elbows to the floor (B).

Modification

If you have knee injuries, avoid this pose. For tight quads, put a bolster under your back.

FINAL RELAXATION

Relax every muscle
in your body.

Stay with the breath.

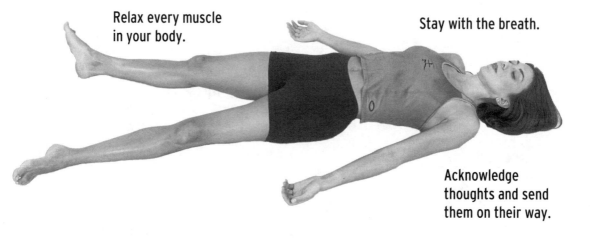

Acknowledge
thoughts and send
them on their way.

FINAL RELAXATION

This pose provides relaxation at the end of every workout.

Getting into the pose

Lie down on your back. Let your arms flop out to the sides. Let your feet roll open.

Holding the pose

Relax. Inhale deeply. Hold. Find peace and calm. Release stress and tension. Keep your attention on the breath.

PART II

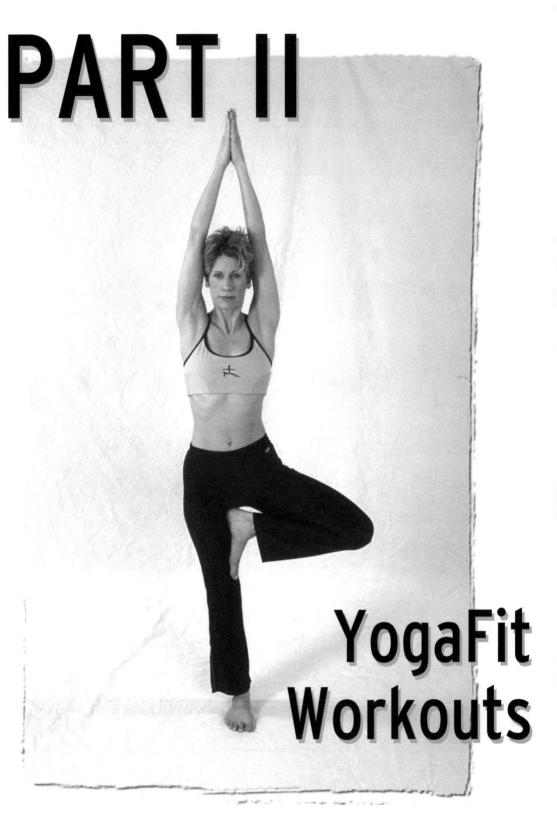

YogaFit
Workouts

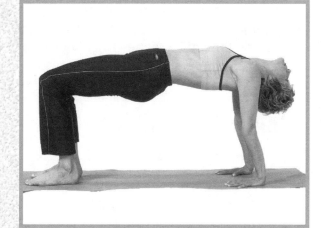

CHAPTER 7

Personalizing a YogaFit Workout

This part of the book will help you assemble the poses introduced in part I to build your own personal YogaFit workout. Select and follow an appropriate class format for your level of expertise and physical condition. Only when you fully understand the concept of a complete YogaFit workout should you start to assemble classes on your own. You should, however, feel free to modify or omit poses that are contraindicated because of a medical condition or because they simply feel uncomfortable. You will feel sensations that might be slightly uncomfortable as the body adjusts to the practice; however, anything that is painful should be avoided.

Important Advice

First and foremost, you should be aware of special conditions such as injuries or pregnancy before you start your workout. Please go back to chapter 1 to read more about YogaFit and special conditions. And always check with your physician when starting this or any other new workout.

Especially in the beginning, it is advisable to follow the class formats in chapters 8, 9, and 10 to get properly acquainted with the YogaFit style. Once you are familiar with the class sequences, you can experiment on new class formats on your own—but don't forget that the YogaFit class formats in this book ensure a total body/mind experience. You will work *all* body parts (legs, arms, torso, sides, shoulders, neck, back, waist, abs, and inner organs). Each class combines standing with seated and lying poses and progresses from a warm-up with heat-building sequences to deep and relaxing stretches and a cool-down. The class formats also ensure that every pose is followed by an appropriate counterpose (e.g., every back bend is followed by a forward bend, and so on).

As you progress in your practice, learn to understand the physical and mental logic of the practice and how it affects your body and mind. Only when you fully comprehend the structure of these classes should you experiment on your own, or you will be cheated out of some of the benefits of YogaFit. In a worst-case scenario, you might even injure yourself (e.g., if you attempted deep stretches before your body had a chance to fully warm up).

Be patient and consistent. YogaFit is best practiced three times a week or more. Make time for your routine; you will soon notice a difference. You will also learn that there is no "bad" or "wrong" YogaFit practice as long as you go at your own pace, breathe, and allow yourself to experience how each pose feels to you at any given moment. Always listen to your body and learn.

Each practice will be a reward in itself. You will feel better without the risk of burning out or getting bored. YogaFit can be your companion for life, and it can help you achieve all of your goals, not just the physical ones.

Before You Start

Familiarize yourself with the poses described in part I. The class formats help you remember, but they are not the full descriptions of the poses and their modifications.

In YogaFit classes we usually hold the poses for three to five breaths. You can extend the time you stay in the poses for a deeper stretch and more intensity (especially during Mountain III), or you can move through the poses with only one or two breaths in the pose for a more cardiovascular workout.

Move controlled and consciously from pose to pose. Observe your body without judgment, and always be aware of when you need to take a break. We suggest that you move into Child's Pose for a few breaths if you need to rest. Listen to your body. Only you know what is good for you on any given day.

Understand that your body will be tight in certain areas and more flexible in others. One side of your body will be more flexible than the other. One side of your body will be stronger than the other. Observe and learn. The YogaFit practice will help you even out some of these imbalances, but each person's body has its own limits.

Be patient. You will most likely be able to accomplish certain poses only after having practiced regularly for a while. In fact, one of the beautiful moments in your YogaFit practice will be the time when you find yourself in a pose that you could not do in previous workouts. But never force a pose, and never push yourself beyond your limits.

Understand that there is always a next step in YogaFit. Even when you have mastered the basic poses, you will always find a new place to go. Ultimately, you should attempt to flow with ease from one pose to another, no matter how invigorating the poses are. And when you find yourself holding one of these challenging poses, know that focused breath can take you through it. Stay calm amidst the storm, smile . . . and breathe.

Here are the YogaFit workouts I will introduce in this book:

YogaFit Classic: A 40-minute workout containing all the basic YogaFit elements. This workout is detailed in chapter 8.

Power YogaFit: A more vigorous 75-minute workout for those who are advanced practitioners of YogaFit in good physical health. Chapter 9 presents this workout.

YogaFit Lite: A 75-minute workout for beginners, pregnant women, those who mostly seek relaxation and restoration, seniors, children, and people with medical conditions. See chapter 10 for YogaFit Lite.

CHAPTER 8

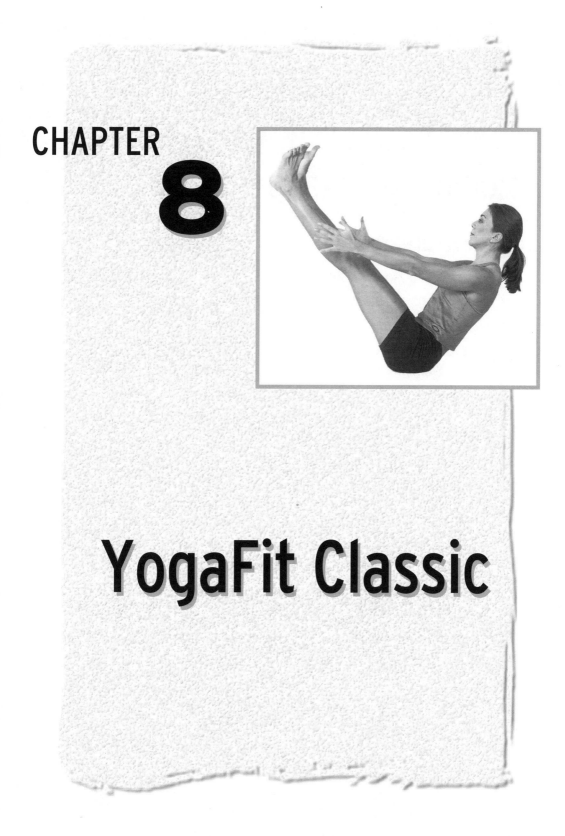

YogaFit Classic

ogaFit Classic is a 40-minute program containing all the basic YogaFit elements. You will get a total body/mind workout in a relatively short amount of time. This is the perfect practice to set up your regular YogaFit routine. This is exactly the same workout as presented on the *Beth Shaw's YogaFit Workout* video (for purchasing information, see the "YogaFit Workout Essentials" section of the introduction to this book, page xvii).

MOUNTAIN I–BREATHING

Deep Breathing

Stand in Mountain Pose
Arms are at your sides or on your midsection
Close eyes
Feel belly extend on inhalation and contract on exhalation
Keep abs tight
Repeat (about 10 breaths)

Forward Fold

Fold upper body forward and down
Bend knees slightly
Hold onto elbows
Close eyes
Shake out the head and relax the neck
Breathe into back of legs and upper back
Sinking breath: Exhale–sink into body
Release elbows
(Stay folded for Chest Expansion)

Chest Expansion

Place arms behind back; interlace fingers
Bring arms over head
Move arms down toward the front
Keep a slight bend in the knees
Release and inhale arms up to the sky

MOUNTAIN I—WARM-UP SERIES

Sunflower

Take a wide stance (feet 3-4 feet apart) and turn sideways on mat
Move both arms up to the sky on an inhalation
On the exhalation bend the knees and lower the arms to the ground
Repeat a few times to warm up the body

Standing Lateral Flexion

Come to front of mat
Stand with feet slightly apart
Bring left arm up; right arm drops
Bend to side (right side)
Slide right arm down right side
On exhalation, sink into pose
Breathe; become aware of how body feels
Switch sides
Modification: Keep the lower arm on your hip

MOUNTAIN II—WORK

Airplane

Bend forward halfway

Keep back flat

Draw arms back with palms facing down

Squeeze shoulder blades together

Draw tailbone back

Keep neck neutral (imagine a beam of light shining ahead from the top of your head)

Modification: Keep arms on hips to protect lower back, and keep a slight bend in your knees

Standing Twist

Start from Forward Fold

Bring left arm down, right arm up

Roll chest open

Look up to right arm

Slightly bend left knee for a deeper twist

Switch arms on exhalation

Modification: Press fist into floor instead of palm

Standing Chest Expansion

Stand

Bring arms behind back

Interlace fingers

Raise arms up

Chair

Stand

Bend knees and lower hips

Lift upper body from the gluteus

Stretch arms out in front; keep elbows soft

Drop shoulders down, away from ears

Hold for five breaths

Fold forward

Come up and reach arms over head

Repeat Chair

Advanced: Balance Chair (go up on your toes)

Hold for five deep breaths

Downward Facing Dog

Move to front of mat

Raise arms

Fold forward

Step feet back

Spread fingers

Press heels down

Relax head and neck

Lift tailbone up to the sky

Push with your palms and heels

Cat-Cow Stretch

Start on hands and knees

Place hands under shoulders

Arch the back; raise the head up (cow)

Round the back; bring the head down (cat)

Keep stomach muscles tight (the work comes from the center—the abs)

Repeat 10 times

Spinal Balance

Start on all fours

Bring left leg and right arm up and straight out

Keep head and neck neutral (crown of the head moves forward)

Keep eyes down

Switch sides

Repeat several times on each side

Extended Child's Pose

Sit back on heels

Bring arms out in front of you

Rest for three breaths

Modification: Bring arms to your sides

Downward Facing Dog

Tuck toes under and push back

Spread fingers

Press heels down

Relax head and neck

Lift tailbone up to the sky

Push back through palms and heels

Plank

Move forward so that hips are level with upper body

Hands are directly under shoulders

Fingers are spread widely

Tighten abs, glutes, and inner thighs

Hold

Modification: Drop knees

ed, "hug" the ribcage

nd

s

h, keeping knees off floor

f the feet

ard

y from ears

and inner thighs tight

Modification: Drop knees and hips for Cobra
Bend knees, look up to hands, softly jump feet up to hands
Modification: Walk feet up to hands
Slowly roll up; bring head up last

Downward Facing Dog

Push back and roll onto your toes
Press through the palms and heels
Lift tailbone
Five breaths
Bend knees, look up to hands, softly jump feet up to hands
Modification: Walk feet up to hands
Inhale arms up and lengthen your body

Back Bend

Stand up straight
Place hands on sacrum
Arch back while lifting torso
Let neck fall back and relax

Standing Forward Fold

Inhale arms up and lower to ground
Bend knees slightly

Monkey

Place fingers in front of feet
Move your chest away from the thighs and look up
Straighten your back as much as possible
Release back into Forward Fold

Plank and Flow Series

Palms on the ground, jump or walk back
Lower down into Crocodile pose
Push back into Downward Facing Dog
Repeat one more time (Plank, Crocodile, Downward Facing Dog)

Warrior I

Step right foot forward
Angle left foot slightly inward
Bend right knee in a 90-degree angle
Keep left leg straight
Press outer edge of left foot into floor
Lift arms, palms facing
Lift chest
Let lower body sink
Hold for five breaths
Straighten right leg and fold upper body over leg

Pyramid

Breathe into hamstring

Place palms on the floor and step back into Downward Facing Dog

Downward Facing Dog

Repeat on other side (Warrior I and Pyramid)

Downward Facing Dog—repeat Warrior I on each side

Flow Series

Downward Facing Dog, Plank, Crocodile, Upward Facing Dog

Repeat this series two more times

Modification: Drop your knees

Downward Facing Dog to Warrior I

Warrior II

Extend arms out to sides

Keep front knee bent

Square hips to the side

Look out over forward hand

Hold

Reverse Warrior

Raise forward hand up to the sky

Drop other hand on back of the straight leg

Make it a side stretch

Back to Warrior II

Placing both hands on floor, move into Downward Facing Dog

Repeat series on opposite side

Warrior I, Warrior II, Reverse Warrior

Flow Series

Downward Facing Dog, Plank, Crocodile, Upward Facing Dog

Repeat this series two more times
Modification: Drop your knees
Hold Downward Facing Dog for five breaths

Pyramid

Step right leg forward and straighten both legs
Back leg is turned in
Inhale arms up and then fold over forward leg
Keep front knee bent if your head does not reach the knee

Triangle

Inhale arms up and bring upper body to center
Keep your feet in alignment
Extend both arms out at shoulder height
Reach forward with your right arm and then drop right hand on right ankle or shin
Reach left arm up to the sky, look up to the hand if comfortable
Keep your body flat
Hold

Reverse Twisting Triangle

Bring left palm down to the inside or outside of right foot
Bring right arm up and twist body open if possible
Hold
Release both arms down to ground

Sun God

Inhale arms up and bring upper body to center

Sink low into hips and extend both arms out to the side, palms face up

Keep spine straight

Hold

Straighten both legs

Triangle on other side

Keep left foot straight, right foot turned in

Extend both arms out at shoulder height

Reach forward with your left arm and then drop left hand on left ankle or shin

Reach right arm up to the sky, look up to the hand if comfortable

Keep your body flat

Hold

Reverse Twisting Triangle

Bring right palm down to inside or outside of left foot

Bring left arm up and twist body open; look up if possible

Hold

Release both arms down to ground

Sun God

Inhale arms up and bring upper body to center

Sink low into hips and extend both arms out to the side, palms face up

Keep spine straight

Hold

Straighten both legs

Standing Straddle Splits

Exhale palms down
Open feet a bit wider
Bring your elbows down if you can
Modification: Palms on the ground

MOUNTAIN III–DEEP AND RELAXING STRETCHES

Extended Child's Pose

Sit back on heels
Bring arms out in front of you
Rest for three breaths
Modification: Bring arms to your sides

Camel

Kneel
Put fists into upper hips
Open chest toward sky, roll shoulders back
Bring head back and relax
Push hips forward
Advanced: Hands move onto heels (toes are tucked under, or, for more intensity, feet are flat on the floor)
Hold for five breaths and then release upper body back up slowly
Modification: Leave fists in sacrum

Extended Child's Pose

Sit back on your heels and extend arms out in front of you

Cobra

Come up on your elbows and push lower body back flat on the ground

Open up chest

Advanced: Press into palms and pull chest higher

Release back down, rest on one cheek for three breaths

Superman

Lie on stomach

Lift both arms and both legs and look up in front of you

Hold

Modification: Bring arms to side

Release back down, rest on other cheek for three breaths

Bow

Bend both knees

Reach back and grab both ankles

Lift chest, push back through your feet to lift higher

Release

Extended Child's Pose

Sit back on your heels and extend arms out in front of you

Seated Forward Fold

Sit off on one side and extend legs

Draw up arms on the inhale

Fold forward on the exhale

Drop the hands on the shins, floor, or feet

Release

Modification: Bend knees if hamstrings are very tight

Boat

Bend knees and lift feet off the floor

Grab on to the back of the knees

Straighten your legs and place your hands at the sides of your hips

If possible, lift arms parallel to the floor

Keep the chest lifting and the stomach muscles strong to support the lower back

Hold and then release legs back to the ground

Modification: Place hands under knees

Tabletop

Bend both knees, soles of the feet are on the ground

Place hands behind back, fingers facing toward feet

Raise hips into a tabletop

Lift the right leg up if you can and cross the right ankle over the left knee

Slowly sink your hips and come to a sitting hip opener

Inhale the right leg back up and then switch legs

Back into hip stretch on other side

Release into a seated position

Butterfly

Soles of the feet come together

Move knees down toward the ground

Press elbows into sides of knees to open them wider (don't force anything)

Slowly fold upper body forward and down

Hold

Lying Down Spinal Twist

Lie on back with both legs straight

Bring right knee into chest, twist to left and move knee toward ground

Extend right arm out to right side; look to right side

Try to keep both shoulders on floor

Place left hand on right knee and move knee closer to ground

Repeat on other side

Knees to Chest

Bring knees to chest

Rock gently from side to side

Bridge

Lie on back

Bend knees, with soles of the feet on the ground about hip-width apart

Arms are at your sides

Push hips up slowly

Advanced: Interlace fingers under your back and walk shoulders in

Modification: Support lower back with hands

Release by slowly rolling down, vertebra by vertebra

Knees to Chest

Rock gently from side to side

Abdominal and Oblique Work (Three-Part Variation)

Lie on back

Bring feet down to floor (knees up)

Interlace hands behind head

Raise upper body straight up on the exhalation

Release on the inhalation

Then move right elbow to left knee on the exhalation

Release on the inhalation

Left elbow to right knee on the exhalation and release on the inhalation

Repeat the three-part abdominal work about 10 times

Advanced: Lift legs straight up

Plough (Optional)

Lie on back

Bring both legs up and over head

Place hands under hips for support

Modification: Bring your legs straight up against a wall

Advanced: Interlace your hands behind your back and walk the shoulders in

Shoulder Stand

Raise your legs up

Support your lower back with your hands

Move elbows closer toward each other

Walk hands farther up back

Keep leg muscles, abs, and glutes very tight

Advanced: Attempt to bring your legs up as straight as possible

Modification: Lie down with your knees bent, hold on to your big toes with the index and middle fingers of each hand and gently press your knees down toward the floor

Plough (Optional)

From Shoulder Stand

Bring feet over head

Grab onto feet or ankles

Roll out slowly

Bring knees into chest

Fish

Lie on back

Bring elbows down under shoulders

Arch back; place top of head on (or move toward) floor

Open heart center

MOUNTAIN III–DEEP RELAXATION

Stretch

Lie on back
Bring arms back; extend overhead
Stretch

Tighten Body

Tighten fists, arms, legs, face, all muscles
Release with a big sigh
Repeat

Corpse Pose, Final Relaxation (5–10 min)

Cover body with towel or blanket, or put on a warm sweater
Lie on back
Roll legs open and turn feet out
Place hands at sides, palms up
Close eyes
Breathe deeply
Let go and feel what's going on in your body
Consciously try to relax one muscle group after another, starting at the feet and working all the way up to your head
If your mind wanders, bring your awareness back to the breath

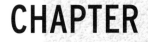

CHAPTER

9

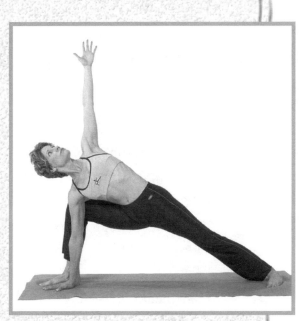

Power YogaFit

ant to step it up a notch? Feeling very energetic today? Longing for a good sweat? Go for 75 minutes of a vigorous workout! Who said that yoga was just a little stretching and meditating? However, I don't want to scare you away—modifications are designed to help you get started and progress to a more advanced level with time.

MOUNTAIN I—BREATHING

Deep Breathing

Stand in Mountain Pose
Place hands on midsection or at your sides
Close eyes
Feel belly extend on inhalation and contract on exhalation
Keep abs tight
Repeat
Modification: Use any other breathing technique from chapter 2

Forward Fold

Fold upper body forward and down
Keep knees bent slightly
Hold onto elbows
Close eyes
Relax neck
Keep a slight bend in your knees
Breathe into back of legs and upper back
Sinking breath: Exhale—sink into body
Release elbows
(Stay folded for Chest Expansion)

Chest Expansion

Bring arms behind back; interlace fingers

Bring arms over head

Move arms down toward the front

Keep knees bent

MOUNTAIN I—WARM-UP SERIES

Sunflower

Take a wide stance (feet 3-4 feet apart) and turn sideways on mat

Move both arms up to the sky on an inhalation

On the exhalation, bend the knees and lower the arms to the ground

Repeat a few times to warm up the body

Standing Lateral Flexion

Come to front of mat

Stand with feet slightly apart

Bring left arm up; drop right arm

Bend to side (right side)

Slide right arm down right side

On exhalation, sink into pose

Switch sides

Modification: Keep one arm on hip

Power YogaFit

MOUNTAIN II—WORK

Airplane

Bend forward halfway

Keep back flat

Keep palms facing down; draw arms back

Squeeze shoulder blades together

Draw tailbone back

Keep neck neutral (imagine a light beam shining ahead from top of head)

Modification: Keep arms on hips to protect lower back

Standing Twist

From Forward Fold

Bring left arm down, right arm up

Roll chest open

Look up to right arm

Slightly bend left knee for a deeper twist

Switch arms on exhalation

Modification: Press fist into floor instead of using palms

Advanced: Bring the lifted arm behind your back

Standing Chest Expansion

Stand

Bring arms behind back

Interlace fingers

Raise arms up

Keep a slight bend in your knees

Chair

Stand

Bend knees and lower hips

Lift upper body from the gluteus

Stretch arms out in front; keep elbows soft

Drop shoulders down, away from ears

Hold for five breaths

Fold forward

Come up and reach arms over head

Repeat Chair three times (deepen each time)

Advanced: Balance Chair (come up on your toes)

Hold for five deep breaths

Release

Forward Fold and Chest Expansion

Fold forward, deeper into hamstrings

Place hands behind back

Interlace fingers

Open shoulders

Release arms

Keep a slight bend in your knees

Downward Facing Dog

Move to front of mat

Raise arms

Fold forward

Step feet back

Spread fingers

Press heels down

Relax head and neck

Point tailbone up to the sky

Push back

Plank

Move hips level with upper body
Place hands directly under shoulders
Spread fingers apart wide
Tighten abs, glutes, and inner thighs
Hold

Crocodile

Lower body slowly and hold 4 inches above ground
Modification: Drop knees

Upward Facing Dog

Slide upper body through while keeping knees off floor
Open chest; gaze forward
Drop shoulders down, away from ears
Keep abs, glutes, and inner thighs tight
Modification: Cobra pose with lower body on the ground
Bend knees; look up to hands; softly jump feet up to hands
Modification: Walk feet up to hands
Inhale your arms up to the sky

Back Bend

Stand up straight
Place hands on sacrum
Arch back while lifting torso
Let neck fall back and relax
Advanced: Let hands slide down hamstrings

Standing Forward Fold

Inhale arms up then bring them down to the ground
Keep a slight bend in your knees

Wrist Stretch

Put hands under feet while bending knees
Slowly straighten legs as much as possible
Stretch upper and lower back
Release, and slowly roll up

Mountain Pose

Stand straight
Keep shoulders, hips, and heels in alignment
Tighten abs; close eyes
Breathe
Check out how you feel

Downward Facing Dog

Raise arms
Fold forward
Step feet back
Spread fingers
Press heels down
Relax head and neck
Point tailbone up to the sky
Push back

Downward Facing Dog (lifted leg)

Lift one leg up in the air; switch legs
Drop to knees

Cat-Cow Stretch

Start on hands and knees

Place hands under shoulders

Arch the back; keep head up (cow)

Round the back; bring head down (cat)

Keep stomach muscles tight (the work comes from the center–the abs)

Repeat 10 times

Spinal Balance

Start on hands and knees

Bring left leg and right arm up and straight out

Keep head and neck neutral (crown of head moves forward)

Keep eyes down

Switch sides

Repeat three times on each side

Child's Pose

Sit back on heels

Bring arms down to sides of body, forehead touches the ground

Rest for three breaths

Variation: Extend your arms out in front of you

(Come back to this resting pose at any time)

Flow Series

Downward Facing Dog, Plank, Crocodile, Upward Facing Dog

Repeat series

Modifications: Drop knees

Sink deeply into Downward Facing Dog; hold for five deep breaths

Bend knees, look up to your hands and jump forward to hands

Inhale arms up over head

Exhale arms down into a Forward Fold

Monkey

Exhale arms down into a Forward Fold

Look up in Monkey pose by moving the chest away from the thighs

Keep back as flat as possible

Release into a Forward Fold

Plank

Walk or jump back into Plank

Kneeling Side Plank

Drop your left knee

With the left hand on the floor, raise the right arm and open the right side of the body

Keep right leg straight

Open the right side of the chest to the sky

Pull energy from the navel center up to the hands

Advanced: Straighten out both legs and balance on the outside edge of the left foot and the inside edge of the right foot

Move back into Plank and switch sides

Flow Series

Downward Facing Dog, Plank, Crocodile, Upward Facing Dog

Modifications: Drop knees

Back to Crocodile, Plank, Upward Facing Dog, Downward Facing Dog

Five breaths in Downward Facing Dog

Camel

Drop knees

Put fists into sacrum

Open chest toward sky

Bring head back and relax

Move slowly into a back bend

Advanced: Hold on to your heels (toes curled under, or for more intensity, feet flat on the floor)

Hold for five breaths

Extended Child's Pose

Sit back on heels with arms extended out in front of you

Downward Facing Dog

Curls your toes under and push back

Push with your palms and heels

Hold for three breaths

Flow Series

Downward Facing Dog, Plank, Crocodile, Upward Facing Dog

Modifications: Drop knees

Back to Crocodile, Plank, Upward Facing Dog, Downward Facing Dog

Five breaths in Downward Facing Dog

Warrior I

Step right foot forward
Angle left foot
Bend right knee in a 90-degree angle
Keep left leg straight
Press outer edge of left foot into floor
Lift arms, palms facing
Bring chest forward and up
Let lower body sink

Pyramid

Straighten forward leg
Fold over forward leg

Standing Straddle Splits

Bring upper body to center
Inhale arms up and exhale them down to the ground
Step feet out as wide as possible
Move crown of head toward floor, lower elbows down if possible
Inhale arms back up

Warrior I on other side

Turn over to the left side
Left foot straight forward
Angle right foot
Bend left knee in a 90-degree angle
Keep right straight
Press outer edge of right foot into floor
Lift arms, palms facing
Bring chest forward and up
Let lower body sink

Pyramid over left leg

Straighten forward leg
Fold over forward leg

Downward Facing Dog

Step back into Downward Facing Dog

Flow Series

Downward Facing Dog, Plank, Crocodile, Upward Facing Dog
Repeat
Modifications: Drop knees
Five breaths in Downward Facing Dog
Downward Facing Dog to Warrior I

Warrior II

Extend arms out to sides
Keep knee bent
Open up body to side (if right leg forward, twist to left)
Look out over forward hand
Hold

Reverse Warrior

Raise forward hand
Lower other hand
Stretch forward hand toward back; keep front knee bent
(This becomes a side stretch)
Back to Warrior II

Extended Angle

Drop right hand inside right foot, stretch left arm up to sky
Advanced: Move upper arm overhead

Flow Series

Plank, Crocodile, Upward Facing Dog, Downward Facing Dog

Both palms come down in front, move into Plank
Modifications: Drop knees
Five breaths in Downward Facing Dog

Repeat series on opposite side

Warrior I, Warrior II, Reverse Warrior, Extended Angle

Flow Series

Downward Facing Dog, Plank, Crocodile, Upward Facing Dog

Modifications: Drop knees
Five breaths in Downward Facing Dog

Pigeon

Lift right leg high up to the sky
Bend the knee and bring the knee into an angled position under body
Lower body down over bent knee
Extend arms out in front
Hold for five breaths
Palms push up upper body, inhale
Curl toes under and push back into Downward Facing Dog on the exhalation
Lift your right leg and shake it out well
Lift left leg up high, bend knee and bring it down under the body
Continue stretch on this side
End in Downward Facing Dog and shake out the left leg

Flow Series

Downward Facing Dog, Plank, Crocodile, Upward Facing Dog

Modifications: Drop knees
Three breaths in Downward Facing Dog

Triangle

Step right leg forward
Turn upper body to center
Extend arms out at shoulder height
Turn right leg out, left leg in
Bring right arm out and down to form triangle
Keep body flat

Reverse Twisting Triangle

Bring left palm down to the inside or outside of right foot
Bring right arm up and twist body open, look up to the hand
Bring both arms down to ground

Balancing Half-Moon

Straighten forward leg, bring back leg up into a 90-degree angle
Keep right hand down, left hand on the left hip
Roll hips open (to left)
Slowly extend the left arm up
If balanced, look up to your left hand
Hold and release

Flow Series

Downward Facing Dog, Plank, Crocodile, Upward Facing Dog

Modifications: Drop knees three to five breaths in Downward Facing Dog

Triangle, Reverse Twisting Triangle, Half-Moon

Repeat on other side

MOUNTAIN III—DEEP AND RELAXING STRETCHES

Downward Facing Dog

Drop knees; lower down to stomach

Cobra

Elbows under shoulders, pull chest up
Advanced: Press into palms and pull chest carefully up

Knot

Lie on stomach
Cross arms under shoulders
Lie down on crossed arms
Hold
Switch arms and hold

Superman

Lie on stomach
Lift arms forward, lift legs, look up, lift chest
Hold
Repeat
Modification: Lift arms to side
(Take a short rest on stomach before Bow)

Bow

Lie on stomach, bend both knees
Reach back and grab ankles with hands
Push back through your ankles and feet
Hold and release

Knees to Chest

Roll over onto back
Bring knees into chest

Spinal Twist

Hold right knee in; move left leg to floor
Bring right knee to left side of body
Keep right shoulder down
Turn head to right
Hold
Switch sides

Bridge

Lie on back
Bring soles down on the ground, feet hip-width apart
Hands are at your sides
Push hips up
Advanced: Interlace hands under back and walk shoulders in
Hold
Modification: Support back with hands
Bring one leg to sky
Switch legs
Release by slowly rolling down, vertebra by vertebra

Knees to Chest

Rock gently from side to side

Abdominal Work

Lie on back
Bring feet down to floor (knees up)
Interlace hands behind head
Raise upper body
Repeat 10 times
Keep hands behind head
Lift legs straight up
Roll up, lifting shoulders off ground
Repeat 10 times

For the Obliques

Bend knees
Raise right shoulder to left knee
Raise left shoulder to right knee
Repeat alternating sides
Modification: Bicycle legs

Bridge, Knees to Chest

Seated Forward Fold

Roll up to seated position
Inhale arms up and exhale them down in front
Drop hands on shins, floor, or feet
Hold and release
Modification: Bend knees if hamstrings are very tight

Boat

Bend knees and lift feet off the floor

Grab on to the back of the knees

Straighten your legs and place your hands at the sides of your hips

If possible, lift arms parallel to the floor

Keep the chest lifting and the stomach muscles strong to support the lower back

Hold and release

Repeat

Modification: Place hands under knees

Incline Plank

Seated position

Place hands behind back, fingers facing toward feet

Raise hips so that body forms a straight plank

Drop head back

Hold

Seated Straddle Splits

Seated position

Spread legs wide apart

Lift arms up over head; fold forward

Keep back as flat as possible

Breathe deeply into pose

Extend arms to front

Move chest toward the ground

Butterfly

Take a seated position

Bring soles of feet together

Move knees out to the sides; press elbows into sides of knees to open them wider (don't force it)

Slowly fold upper body forward and down

Hold for 10 breaths

Seated Twist

From a seated position, extend the legs out

Bring the right knee up with the sole of the foot on the floor

Place the left elbow outside the right knee, and twist the body at the waist

Twist further on every exhalation

Repeat on other side

Knees to Chest

Roll back and bring knees to chest

Plough (Optional)

Lie on back

Bring both legs up and over head

Place hands under hips for support

Modification: Move legs only as far toward ground as you can; support lower back with hands

Advanced: If your toes reach the ground, interlace your hands behind the back and walk your shoulders in

Shoulder Stand

Raise your legs up
Support your lower back with your hands
Move elbows closer toward each other
Walk hands farther up back
Keep leg muscles, abs, and glutes very tight
Advanced: Attempt to bring your legs up as straight as possible

Plough (Optional)

From Shoulder Stand
Bring feet over head
Grab onto feet or ankles
Roll out slowly
Bring knees into chest

Fish

Lie on back
Bring elbows down under shoulders
Arch back
Place top of head on (or move toward) floor
Open heart center
(Counterpose for inversion)

MOUNTAIN III–DEEP RELAXATION

Stretch

Lie on back
Bring arms back; extend overhead
Stretch

Tighten Body

Tighten fists, arms, legs, face, all muscles
Release and repeat

Corpse Pose, Final Relaxation (5–10 min)

Cover body with towel or blanket, or put on a warm sweater
Lie on back
Roll legs open, turn feet out
Let arms lie by sides, palms up
Close eyes and breathe deeply
Let go and feel body sensations
Consciously try to relax one muscle group after another, starting at the feet and bringing the awareness all the way up to the head
If your mind starts to wander, just bring it back to the breath

Power YogaFit

CHAPTER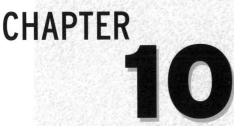

10

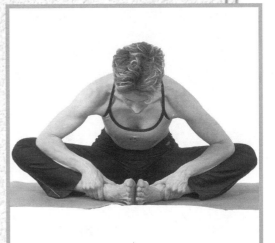

YogaFit Lite

his is the perfect workout if you are just starting with YogaFit, if you are feeling tired, or if you are looking for relaxation. In this 75-minute class, you can also focus more on proper alignment, so it is a good idea to come back to this workout from time to time, even if you prefer the other workouts for your routine. I recommend this class also for pregnant women, seniors, children, and people with medical conditions.

MOUNTAIN I—BREATHING

Deep Breathing

Stand in Mountain Pose

Place hands on midsection or at your sides

Close eyes

Feel belly extend on inhalation and contract on exhalation

Keep abs tight

Repeat

Modification: Use any other breathing technique from chapter 2

Forward Fold

Fold upper body forward and down

Keep knees bent at all times

Hold onto elbows

Close eyes

Relax neck

Breathe into back of legs and upper back

Sinking breath: Exhale–sink into body

Release elbows

(Stay folded for Chest Expansion)

Chest Expansion

Place arms behind back; interlace fingers

Bring arms over head

Move arms down toward the front

Keep knees bent at all times

Modification: Use straps or towel if shoulders are tight

MOUNTAIN I—WARM-UP SERIES

Sunflower

Take a wide stance (feet 3-4 feet apart) and turn sideways on mat

Move both arms up to the sky on an inhale

On the exhale bend the knees and lower the arms to the ground

Repeat a few times to warm up the body

Standing Lateral Flexion

Come to front of mat

Stand with feet slightly apart

Bring left arm up; right arm is on hip

Bend to side (right side)

On exhalation, sink into pose

Switch sides

MOUNTAIN II—WORK

Standing Twist

Start from Forward Fold

Bring left arm down and right arm up

Roll chest open

Look up to right arm

Slightly bend left knee for deeper twist

Switch arms on exhalation

Modification: Press fist into floor instead of using palms

Standing Chest Expansion

Start from Forward Fold

Bring arms behind back

Knees are bent slightly

Interlace fingers

Hold and release

Chair

Inhale up into standing

Bend knees and lower hips

Stretch arms out in front; keep elbows soft

Drop shoulders down, away from ears

Hold for five breaths

Fold forward

Repeat Chair three times (deepen each time)

Release back into Forward Fold

Downward Facing Dog

Walk legs back
Spread fingers
Press heels down
Relax head and neck
Point tailbone up to the sky
Push back
Modification: Drop knees

Plank

Move chest forward into a Plank
Place hands directly under shoulders
Spread fingers wide
Modification: Drop knees

Modified Crocodile

Drop knees, chest, and chin just above the floor with buttocks up in the air
Place hands directly under shoulders
Spread fingers widely
Tighten abs, glutes, and inner thighs
Hold

Cobra

Elbows come down, slide upper body through
Keep elbows on floor
Open chest; gaze forward
Drop shoulders down, away from ears
Keep abs, glutes, and inner thighs tight
Curl toes under and push into downward facing dog pose
Hold for five breaths
Modification: Drop knees

YogaFit Lite

Back Bend

Walk legs up to hands
Inhale arms up over head
Place hands on upper hips
Let neck fall back and relax
Move chest slowly up and back
Don't compress lower back

Standing Forward Fold

Inhale arms up overhead and then fold forward
Bend knees

Monkey

Fingers in front, chest moves away from thighs
Flatten back as much as possible
Release back into Forward Fold
Repeat

Mountain Pose

Inhale arms up overhead
Keep shoulders, hips, and heels in alignment
Keep abs tight and eyes closed
Breathe

Forward Fold

Monkey pose
Forward Fold

Downward Facing Dog

Walk back into Downward Facing Dog

Spread fingers and press palms, keep hands and wrists completely parallel

Press heels down

Relax head and neck

Point tailbone up to the sky

Let chest sink toward the floor

Hold for five breaths

Drop to knees

Cat-Cow Stretch

Start on hands and knees

Place hands under shoulders

Arch the back and bring head up (cow) on the inhalation

Round the back and bring head down (cat) on the exhalation

Keep stomach muscles tight (the work comes from the center–the abs)

Repeat 10 times

Spinal Balance

Start on all fours

Bring left leg and right arm up and straight out

Keep head and neck neutral (crown of head moves forward)

Keep eyes down

Switch sides

Repeat three times on each side

Sunbird

Start on all fours

Move right knee toward forehead on the exhalation

Straigthen the same leg out behind you and up on the inhalation

Arch the back and look up

Keep hips squared to the ground

Repeat a few times and then switch sides

Child's Pose

Sit back on heels

Bring arms down to sides of body

Rest for five breaths

(Come back to this resting pose at any time)

Kneeling Side Stretch

Start on knees

Bring arms up

Drop left arm; put left palm on floor

Stretch right arm up to the sky

Stretch right leg out straight toward right side; keep left knee on floor

Stretch your right side

Pull hip bone forward

Breathe deeply into rib cage

Hold

Switch sides

Hold

Child's Pose

Stay in Child's Pose for three breaths

Camel

Kneel
Put fists back onto upper hips
Open chest up and back
Bring head back and relax if comfortable
Don't compress lower back
Hold for five breaths

Child's Pose

Hold for five breaths
Curl toes under and push up into Downward Facing Dog pose

Downward Facing Dog

Hold for three deep breaths

Warrior I

Step right foot forward
Angle left foot
Bend right knee in a 90-degree angle
Keep left leg straight
Press outer edge of left foot into floor
Lift arms, palms facing
Bring chest forward and up
Let lower body sink

Pyramid

Straighten forward leg
Fold over forward leg

Downward Facing Dog

Go deeper into pose

Repeat series on other side

Warrior I, Pyramid

Downward Facing Dog to Warrior I

Warrior II

Extend arms out to the sides
Keep knee bent
Open up body to side (if right leg is forward, twist to left)
Look out over forward hand
Hold

Reverse Warrior

Raise forward hand
Lower other hand
Stretch forward hand toward back; keep front knee bent
(This becomes a side stretch)
Back to Warrior II
Downward Facing Dog, Child's Pose

Repeat series on other side

Downward Facing Dog, Warrior I, Warrior II, Reverse Warrior

Downward Facing Dog, Child's Pose

Flow Series

Downward Facing Dog, Plank, Crocodile, Upward Facing Dog, Downward Facing Dog

Modification: Drop knees

Child's Pose

Stay in Child's Pose for five breaths

Curl toes under and push up into Downward Facing Dog

Pigeon

Lift right leg high up to the sky

Bend the knee and bring the knee into an angled position under body

Lower body down over bent knee

Extend arms out in front

Hold for five breaths

Palms push up upper body, inhale

Curl toes under and push back into Downward Facing Dog on the exhalation

Lift your right leg and shake it out well

Lift left leg up high, bend knee and bring it down under the body

Continue stretch on this side

End in Downward Facing Dog and shake out the left leg

Triangle

Step right leg forward

Turn upper body to center

Extend arms out at shoulder height

Turn right leg out, left leg in

Bring right arm out and down to form triangle

Keep body flat

Forward Fold, Monkey

Step feet together and inhale arms up–Forward Fold
Look up for Monkey and Forward Fold again
Step back into Downward Facing Dog

Triangle

Triangle over left leg
Come back to Forward Fold, Monkey, and Forward Fold
Walk back into Downward Facing Dog
Drop knees and lie on stomach

MOUNTAIN III–DEEP AND RELAXING STRETCHES

Superman

Lie on stomach
Lift upper torso, legs, and arms (forward)
Hold
Repeat
Modification: Bring arms to sides

Cobra

Slide upper body through into a back bend
Keep elbows on floor
Open chest up; gaze forward
Drop shoulders down, away from ears
Keep abs, glutes, and inner thighs tight

Knees to Chest

Roll over onto back

Bring knees into chest

(Counterpose to the cobra or back bend)

Lying Down Spinal Twist

Hold right knee in; move left leg to floor

Bring right knee to left side of body

Keep right shoulder down

Turn face to right

Hold

Switch sides

Bridge

Lie on back

Bring knees up, feet are on the ground about hip-width apart

Arms are down by your sides

Hold

Release by slowly rolling down, vertebra by vertebra

Repeat

Knees to Chest

Rock gently from side to side

Abdominal Work

Lie on back
Bring feet down to floor (knees up)
Interlace hands behind head
Raise upper body
Repeat 10 times
Keep hands behind head
Lift legs straight up
Roll up, lifting shoulders off ground
Repeat 10 times

For the Obliques

Bend knees
Raise right shoulder to left knee
Raise left shoulder to right knee
Repeat, alternating sides
Modification: Do bicycle motion with feet

Knees to Chest

Bring knees to chest
Roll gently from side to side
(Counterpose to abdominal work)
Roll up to seated position

Seated Forward Fold

Inhale arms up and exhale them down in front
Drop hands on shins, floor, or feet
Hold and release
Modification: Bend knees if hamstrings are very tight

Tabletop

Start in a seated position

Bend knees and place the soles of the feet on the floor, about hip-width apart

Place hands behind back with fingers facing toward feet

Push hips up into a tabletop position

Let head drop back and release

Hold

Release and repeat

Seated Straddle Splits

Seated position

Spread legs wide apart

Lift arms over head and fold forward

Keep back as flat as possible

Breathe deeply into pose

Extend arms in front of you; move chest toward the ground

Butterfly

Start from a seated position

Bring soles of feet together and move knees out to the sides

Press elbows into sides of knees to open them up wider (don't force)

Slowly fold upper body forward and down

Hold for 10 breaths

YogaFit Lite

Seated Twist

From a seated position, extend legs out
Bring right knee up with sole of foot on the floor
Place left elbow outside right knee, and twist body at waist
Twist further on every exhalation
Repeat on other side

Knees to Chest

Roll down and bring knees to chest

Legs against wall

Move mat near a wall
Lift legs and rest them against wall
Move sitting bones as close to wall as possible
Spread legs or keep them closed
Hold for 15 deep breaths

Fish

Lie on back
Bring elbows down under shoulders
Arch back and place top of head on (or move toward) floor
Open heart center

MOUNTAIN III—DEEP RELAXATION

Stretch

Lie on back
Bring arms back and extend over head
Stretch

Tighten body

Tighten fists, arms, legs, face, all muscles

Release

Repeat

Corpse Pose, Final Relaxation (5–10 min)

Cover body with towel or blanket, or put on a warm sweater

Lie on back

Feet turn out

Bring hands to the sides, palms up

Close eyes and breathe deeply

Let go and feel what's going on in your body

Consciously try to relax one muscle group after another, starting at the feet and working all the way up to your head

If your mind wanders, bring your awareness back to the breath

YogaFit Lite

CHAPTER

11

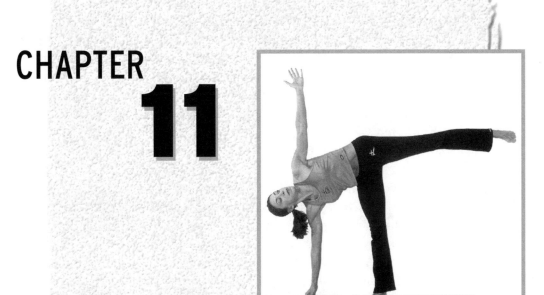

YogaFit for Sports

ogaFit was specifically designed for athletes and people interested in getting a good, total body/mind workout. Because I myself was an athlete first, I understood what yoga could add to any fitness routine and what the best way to incorporate yoga into any practice was.

Traditional exercise programs often overwork certain muscle groups or build muscle bulk unevenly. YogaFit can be extremely helpful in counteracting some of the negative effects these traditional programs have on our bodies.

If you are a weightlifter, you may have noticed that your flexibility levels are severely limited by pumping iron. A rather simple stretch such as a chest expansion might be difficult for you, or you might have to use a shoulder strap because you cannot reach your hands behind your back. A regular YogaFit workout of three 45-to-60-minute sessions per week (or more) can drastically reduce this inflexibility. YogaFit poses are designed to strengthen the muscles by lengthening them, not by creating more bulk.

Bikers and indoor stationary cyclists get a very unbalanced workout of the lower body only. YogaFit works all major muscles groups and combines strength building with cardiovascular conditioning. By moving faster through the flow series, you get more cardiovascular exercise. By holding the poses longer, you can focus more on the strength-building benefits.

Swimming (not listed in the following pages) is a highly recommended total body workout that perfectly combines with a yoga workout. It's great for developing breathing patterns.

A regular YogaFit workout keeps the muscles limber and active without lactic acid buildup. You might say that a regular YogaFit practice "greases" your muscles and connective tissue, which helps prevent injuries and chronic pain.

As an athlete, you can select the most beneficial YogaFit stretches and poses to balance out the effects your sport has on your body. In addition to your YogaFit practice, you should complement your sports practice with these stretches by either using them between weightlifting sets or before and after your workout or training. The following pages list the YogaFit stretches that are the best counterposes for different sports.

RUNNING

Problems: Tight hips, quads, and hamstrings; back pain. Running causes an imbalance in the body because it does not work the upper body. **Focus:** Breath (deep breathing; nose breathing for a more intense, focused workout).

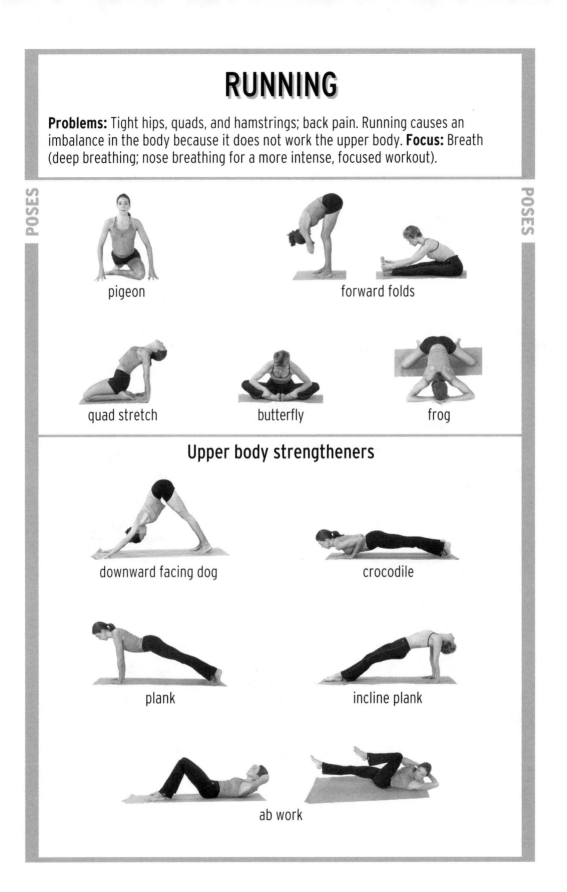

pigeon

forward folds

quad stretch

butterfly

frog

Upper body strengtheners

downward facing dog

crocodile

plank

incline plank

ab work

CYCLING

Problems: Tight hips, quads, and hamstrings; back pain. Cycling and indoor stationary cycling cause an imbalance in the body because they do not work the upper body. The upper body is contracted. **Focus:** Breath (deep breathing; nose breathing for a more intense, focused workout).

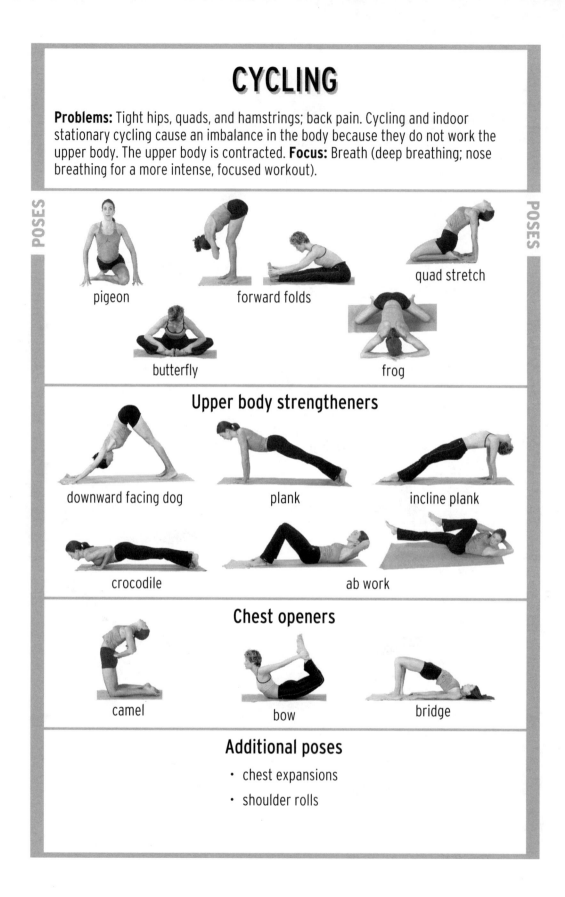

POSES

pigeon

forward folds

quad stretch

butterfly

frog

Upper body strengtheners

downward facing dog

plank

incline plank

crocodile

ab work

Chest openers

camel

bow

bridge

Additional poses

- chest expansions
- shoulder rolls

GOLF AND TENNIS

Problems: Tight hips, quads, and hamstrings; back pain; need for increased range of motion. **Focus:** Concentration (mental aspects; meditation).

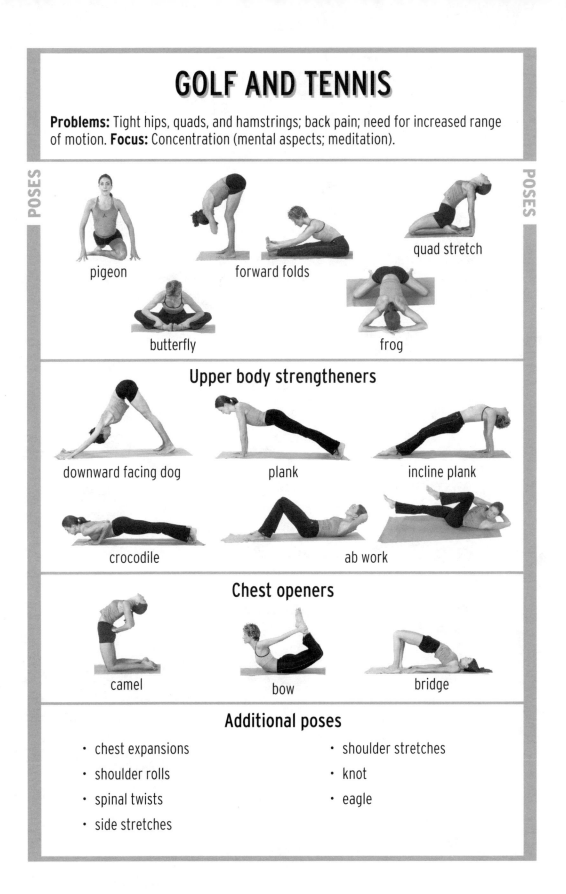

pigeon

forward folds

quad stretch

butterfly

frog

Upper body strengtheners

downward facing dog

plank

incline plank

crocodile

ab work

Chest openers

camel

bow

bridge

Additional poses

- chest expansions
- shoulder rolls
- spinal twists
- side stretches

- shoulder stretches
- knot
- eagle

BASEBALL

Problems: Tight hips, quads, and hamstrings; back pain. Baseball requires a flexible torso. **Focus:** Concentration (mental aspects; meditation).

POSES

POSES

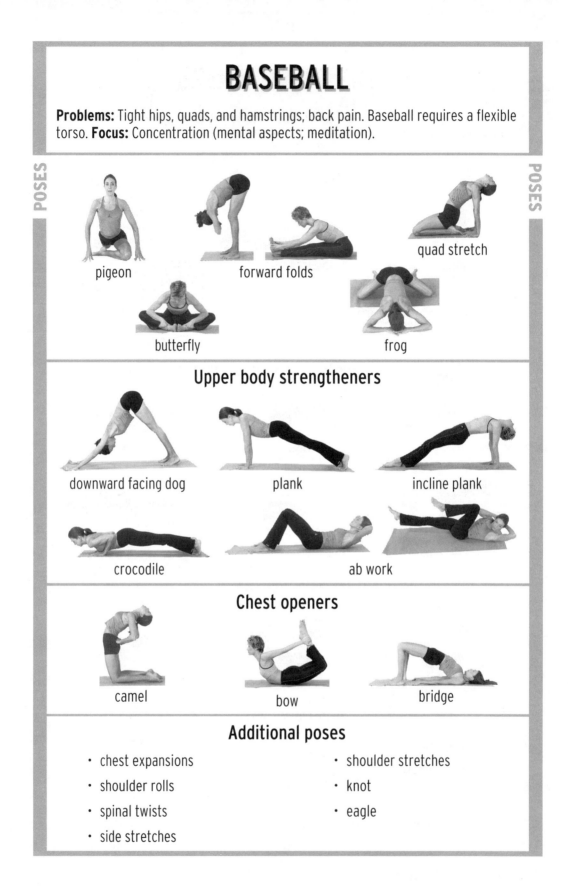

pigeon

forward folds

quad stretch

butterfly

frog

Upper body strengtheners

downward facing dog

plank

incline plank

crocodile

ab work

Chest openers

camel

bow

bridge

Additional poses

- chest expansions
- shoulder rolls
- spinal twists
- side stretches

- shoulder stretches
- knot
- eagle

VOLLEYBALL AND BASKETBALL

Problems: Tight shoulders, hips, quads, and hamstrings; back pain and knee injuries. Needs flexible shoulders. **Focus:** Breath (deep breathing; nose breathing).

Shoulder stretches

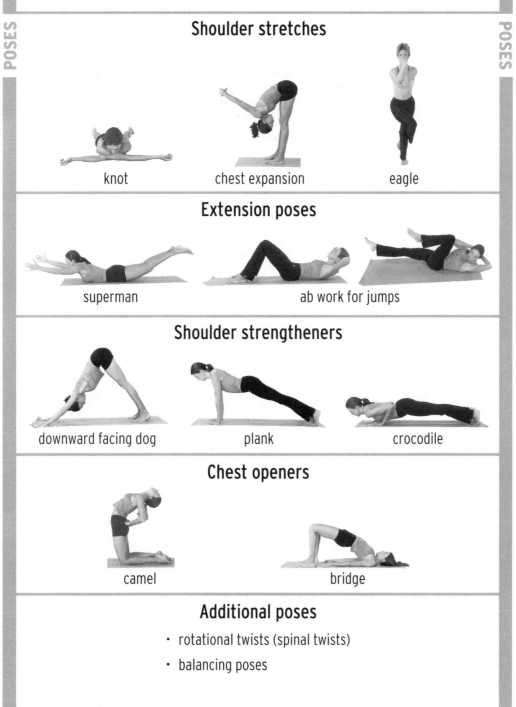

knot

chest expansion

eagle

Extension poses

superman

ab work for jumps

Shoulder strengtheners

downward facing dog

plank

crocodile

Chest openers

camel

bridge

Additional poses

- rotational twists (spinal twists)
- balancing poses

SKIING AND SNOWBOARDING

Problems: Tight hips, ligaments, quads, and hamstrings; back pain. Good balance is a necessity. **Focus:** Breath (deep breathing; nose breathing for a more intense, focused workout).

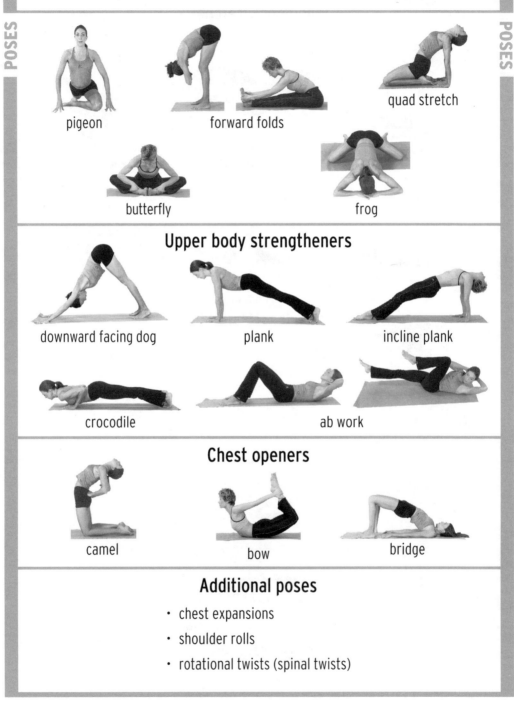

pigeon

forward folds

quad stretch

butterfly

frog

Upper body strengtheners

downward facing dog

plank

incline plank

crocodile

ab work

Chest openers

camel

bow

bridge

Additional poses

- chest expansions
- shoulder rolls
- rotational twists (spinal twists)

WEIGHTLIFTING

Problems: Tight shoulders and leg muscles; back pain. **Focus:** Breath (one breath for every movement).

Note: Weightlifting and yoga can work against each other. Weightlifting shortens and bulks the muscles, whereas yoga lengthens and straightens the muscles. You can still lift weights, but your yoga workout will be more challenging.

Between sets

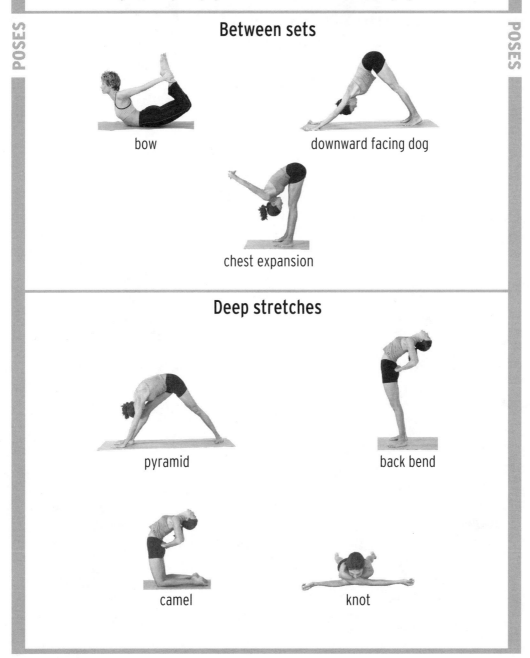

bow

downward facing dog

chest expansion

Deep stretches

pyramid

back bend

camel

knot

KICKBOXING AND BOXING

Problems: Tight shoulders and hips, back pain, and knee problems. **Focus:** Breath (one breath for every movement).

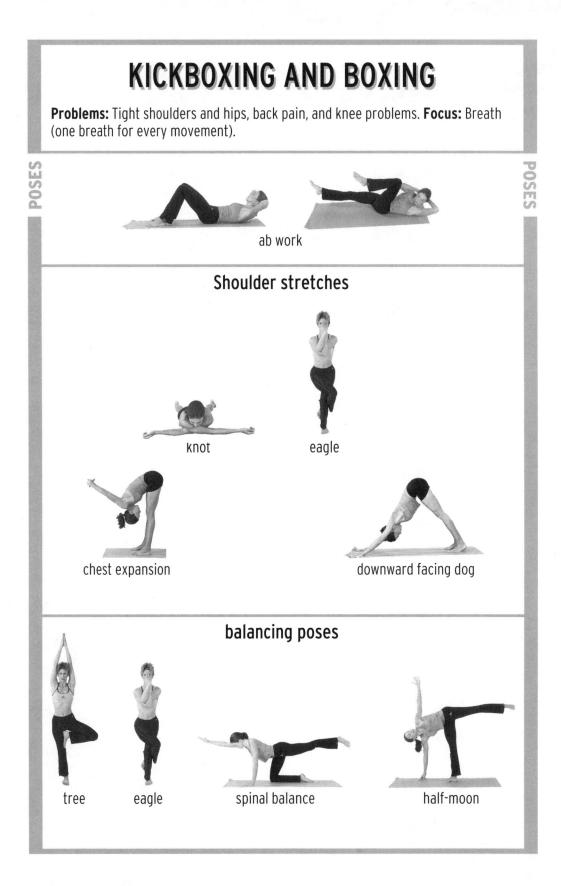

ab work

Shoulder stretches

knot

eagle

chest expansion

downward facing dog

balancing poses

tree   eagle

spinal balance

half-moon

APPENDIX A

YogaFit Teacher Training and Partnering Program

ogaFit offers a Teacher Training Program at two levels to people from the health and fitness industry. If you are a fitness instructor, participating in the program is a great way to further your career and generate additional income. Yoga is the biggest fitness trend of the new millennium; become part of the wave!

The YogaFit Teacher Training Program is the only IHRSA (International Health, Racquet and Sportsclub Association), ACE (American Council on Exercise) and AFAA (Aerobics and Fitness Association of America) certified yoga teacher training program, and training classes are held in numerous locations throughout the United States and other countries. For updated training dates and locations, please visit **www.yogafit.com**, or call toll-free 888-786-3111.

The YogaFit Teacher Training is typically a weekend program of quality, hands-on instruction, team teaching, and enough support material to allow you to start your first yoga class right away. A high-quality yoga mat is included in the Level I Training. For more details and prices, please contact YogaFit.

If your fitness club staff are interested in training, you can contact us, and we will come to you to train your people. Please be aware, however, that participating in the YogaFit Teacher Training Program does not automatically allow you to use the YogaFit name and logo, both of which are international trademarks.

YogaFit offers a Partnering Program that includes teacher training sessions at your facility and marketing materials to promote your YogaFit classes. Only licensees are allowed to use the name YogaFit for their classes. Additional income can be generated by selling YogaFit merchandise, such as YogaFit clothing, music CDs, and mats as well as *Beth Shaw's YogaFit Workout* video and this book. This is an easy, one-step process to starting a YogaFit Partnering Program at your facility immediately. Contact YogaFit for more details at **info@yogafit.com** or toll-free at 888-786-3111.

Recommended Reading, Viewing, and Shopping

Your local or online bookstore features many yoga books, videos, Web sites, and magazines. Here are some of our favorites:

Videos

Beth Shaw's YogaFit Workout. As the companion to this book, the video walks you through the YogaFit Classic workout. To order, call YogaFit at 888-786-3111 or 310-798-8773, or purchase online at **www.yogafit.com**. You can also contact Human Kinetics at **www.humankinetics.com**, or check your local or online bookstore.

Music CDs

YogaFit has compiled music specifically designed for your personal YogaFit workout or class. Descriptions of the poses to move along with these smooth grooves give you an easy start into a great body/mind adventure. To order, call YogaFit at 888-786-3111 or 310-798-8773, or purchase online at **www.yogafit.com**.

Web Sites

YogaFit, at **www.yogafit.com**, offers information about the YogaFit studio in Hermosa Beach, California; teacher trainings worldwide; and the YogaFit licensing program. Plus, you can shop online for clothing, mats, music, videos, books, and more.

Human Kinetics, at **www.humankinetics.com**, offers a wide variety of fitness, sports, and health-related books and videos that can be ordered online.

Conscious Media, at **www.consciousmedia.com**, convinced us with their great selection of body/mind publications and products at great discount prices for online shoppers.

About the Author

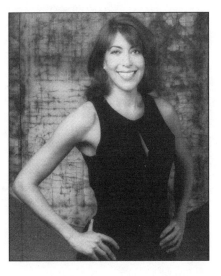

Beth Shaw, president and founder of YogaFit® Training Systems Worldwide, Inc., is recognized throughout the United States and Europe as one of the leading experts in fitness today. She also stars in her own exercise video, *Beth Shaw's YogaFit Workout*.

Her accomplishments don't stop there. She is also an award-winning producer of YogaFit TV and has been published in numerous consumer and fitness publications including *SHAPE, Ahtletic Business, Fitness, The Yoga Journal, CBI, Fitness Product News, Recreation Resources, IDEA Today,* and *LA Parent.*

With 15 years of experience in fitness training and 11 years of yoga practice, Shaw has received teacher certifications from Yoga White Lotus Foundation, Integrative Yoga Therapy Association, Institute of Psycho-Structural Balancing, and Reebok University. She has also completed coursework in the UCLA Fitness Instructors Certification Program. She holds a bachelor of science degree in health marketing from Long Island University.

Shaw founded YogaFit in 1994 and opened her own signature studio in Hermosa Beach, California, in 1998. Her studio presently serves more than 2,000 students a month. Offering an ACE-, AFAA-, and IHRSA-approved teacher training program, thousands of fitness instructors from across the U.S. and Europe have been trained by YogaFit in the last three years.

When not teaching and lecturing internationally, Shaw enjoys reading and taking long bike rides along the beach. She resides in Hermosa Beach, California.

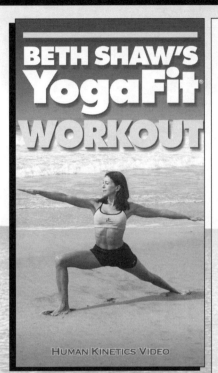
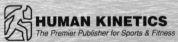